How To Control Your Alcohol Consumption

Learn To Drink Responsibly
So That You Can Enjoy A
Drink
Rather Than Depend On It

Jason Newman

By reading this document, the reader agrees that under no circumstances is the author responsible for any losses, direct or indirect, that are incurred as a result of the use of the information contained within this document, including, but not limited to, errors, omissions, or inaccuracies.

Table of Contents

Introduction

"Drunkenness is nothing but voluntary madness."—**Seneca**

Alcohol is the most socially acceptable drug on the market and the most accessible for almost anyone, regardless of age. Three-quarters of all adults drink. Of those who do drink, 70% are employed, losing their collective companies $81 billion in lost profits due to addiction-related problems. These problems can be anything from injuries to loss of productivity, either by excessive absences or an inability to function.

Excessive drinking accounts for 29% of all traffic fatalities in any given year. Additionally, alcohol is recognized as the cause of six different types of cancer. In the United States, alcohol accounts for $252 billion spent annually. All of these statistics should be alarming and will hopefully afford a moment of thought about your own drinking habits, dear reader.

If you are reading this book, it is highly likely that you want to cut back on your drinking. Perhaps you have friends or family who pushed this book into your hands. The good news: This book is about control, not quitting. Even reducing your alcohol intake by half can lead to improvements in your health, finances, and livelihood. But the first thing to consider is where you are at right now. Do you want to cut down drinking for your health or to help your wallet? Is a job, your marriage, or your kids suffering? Consider how much you drink in a given week.

One of the most shocking facts most people try to ignore is the size of an actual drink. A standard drink in the United States contains 0.6 ounces or 1.2 tablespoons of pure alcohol. Twelve fluid ounces of beer (5% alcohol content), eight ounces of malt liquor (7% alcohol content), five fluid ounces of wine (12% alcohol content), and an ounce and a half of 80-proof spirits (40% alcohol content) are all defined as a single drink. This means a six pack of 18-ounce beer cans is actually nine standard drinks. Very few people actually realize how quickly the math adds up until they work it out for themselves. This can lead to more embarrassment or shock for those who may not realize just how much alcohol they were actually consuming.

Healthy amounts of alcohol, if a person must drink, are one standard-sized drink per day for women and two per day for men, using the measurements above. With the wide variety of alcohol percentages in different drinks and the different types of drinks available, it's no wonder so many people end up drinking more than they mean to. Mixed drinks often contain more alcohol than people think since each shot and a half of spirits equals one standard drink. Something with many types of alcohol mixed in could be at least three or four drinks all on its own.

One of the most important things to know might be how much you spend on alcohol. There are many alcoholics who wind up quitting after they realize the financial hit their habit is costing them. A conservative estimate for cheap beer or wine might be $5 per standard unit—a six pack, a single bottle, etc. If you buy one every night, that's $35 per week and $1,820 per year. Though this can be a shocking wake-up call for some, it is important to be honest with yourself about the addiction or habits that have built up around your drinking. Without knowing these in plenty of detail, your chances of successfully cutting back drop considerably. If you are honest with yourself, your family, and your friends, you can set up the support you need to control your alcohol consumption rather than letting it control you.

Consumption: How Much Is Too Much?

The subject of whether or not to drink can be a touchy one at times. There are some people who simply should not drink: those under the age as allowed by the law (21 in the U.S.); women who are pregnant or trying to become pregnant; those taking medication, whether prescribed or over the counter, that may not interact well with alcohol; people who are performing tasks that require focus, concentration, and alertness (i.e., driving); or recovering alcoholics, just to name a few. In general, if you have trouble saying no or otherwise controlling how much alcohol you are putting in your body, you should abstain if you are able. There are many more dangerous behaviors around alcohol consumption, such as binge drinking or heavy drinking, that should not be common practice.

Binge drinking generally involves ingesting a large amount of alcohol in a short period of time. It is common at bars, parties, and other heavily social interactions where alcoholic drinks are present. This type of behavior is seen more in younger drinkers, especially college students or those who recently came of legal drinking age. Binge drinking is identified as four or more drinks in a single occasion for women and five or more for men. Remember that a standard drink is not measured by the number of glasses one touches, but by the amount of alcohol contained in each drink.

Heavy drinking, more commonly seen among alcoholics, is defined as eight or more drinks per week for women and 15 or more drinks per week for men. The thing that makes heavy drinking such a concern is its tendency to sneak up on a person. Nobody sets out to drink up to a dozen beers per week.

It happens slowly as tolerance builds and often happens without the person even realizing. One night, you get buzzed off of just two glasses of wine or cans of beer. A week later, it may take three. Two weeks after that, you need four. Maybe in the next month, you need a drink to relax before bed.

Alcoholism is a slow progression, a steady increase that few people deliberately plan, and it can grow out of control in apparently no time at all. One way to keep this problem from multiplying uncontrollably is to place limits on how much you can drink in a given day. You can also add stipulations to when or where you are allowed to drink or, perhaps, how you are allowed to pay for your drinks. The introduction of a few easy rules and a modicum of self-control can help an unexpected alcoholic to take a few steps back from the metaphorical ledge. That is a fantastic first step towards cutting back.

Why This Book?

How To Control Your Alcohol Consumption is not about quitting drinking, nor does it advocate quitting without any kind of cutting back on your intake, known as quitting cold turkey. Instead, this book presents the facts about alcohol, its effects on the body, and its addictive properties, as well as tips and tricks to help you cut back on the amount you are drinking and methods to negate some withdrawal effects. Over 30% of people who try to quit drinking will return to it within their first year of trying to quit. By cutting back instead, you will increase your chances of eventual success in quitting completely, as well as increasing the amount of control you have on your current addiction.

This book and its author are not responsible for any decisions readers may make, nor are they responsible for any unsuccessful results readers may have. Some of the choices this book will encourage should steer you toward cutting back on your drinking habit. Even dropping one drink per day can make a tremendous difference. Remember, before you can succeed at any endeavor, you have to put in the effort and try.

Oftentimes, trying can be enough to reach your goal. It can also be helpful to remember why you want to cut back. Has a friend or family member expressed concern? Has your alcohol consumption caused less contact with family or friends? Perhaps you are spending money you don't have in order to get alcohol. This can lead to things like credit card debt or drinking less safe alcohol containing products.

There is a surprising number of household items that contain alcohol in some form and the liver metabolizes them the same way it would beer or wine. These include things like mouthwash, cough syrup, or flavored extracts used for cooking. Drinking these items, especially in large amounts, can be exceedingly dangerous. This leads to the first obvious effect alcohol can have on someone with a severe addiction: hurting the body.

Additionally, excessive drinking can cause changes in mood and temperament. It can severely alter a person's ability to function, preventing them from completing simple tasks such as daily chores or caring for kids or for themselves. Whatever reason you have for wanting to cut back your alcohol intake, please remember that reason and hold tight to it. Remembering why you want to cut back and focusing on how much better your future will be can be a tremendous help in this endeavor.

To everyone trying to cut back their alcohol intake, take it one day at a time and forgive yourself for any setbacks. You can do this. Alcohol does not have to control you any longer. Decreasing your regular intake will give you back control and allow you to reclaim your life.

Chapter 1: Alcohol and Your Body

"Alcohol is an allergy of the body and an obsession of the mind."—**Rita Mae Brown**

Alcohol has a wide variety of effects on the human body, and drinking alcohol affects every part of the body in one way or another. As the second most widely used substance, just after tobacco, it's no wonder we have so much knowledge of this damage. Though the long-term effects are usually given a lot of attention, drinking alcohol also has short-term effects. The most obvious short-term effect would be a hangover.

Hangovers cause issues such as sensitivity to light, nausea, vomiting, diarrhea, and extreme dehydration among other things. Drinking alcohol can cause dramatic shifts in the body's sugar levels, leading to issues such as hypoglycemia. This is caused by the sugar levels dropping very quickly as the alcohol, which is very high in sugar, gets metabolized. Further nausea, dizziness, and headaches caused by low blood sugar can make a hangover even worse.

Drinking disrupts many of the neural pathways in the brain, especially those that deal with communication. This means that different areas of the brain cannot communicate effectively after someone has started to drink. A lack of communication in the brain leads to slower reflexes, less coordination, and trouble communicating with others. Poor decision making happens when the brain can't effectively send messages as needed.

Too much alcohol also has an effect on sleep. Though many people think that drinking can help them get to sleep, this is not true. In fact, drinking can lead to poor quality sleep.

Rather than allowing for rapid eye movement (REM) sleep, which is what allows our bodies to rest, adding alcohol depresses the nervous system. As a result, though someone may fall asleep faster, they do not stay asleep.

Instead of REM sleep, which should happen late in the sleep cycle, the body is more likely to stay in non-REM sleep. Non-REM sleep causes a person to wake up more often and more easily. Getting to sleep while intoxicated is also difficult. Though drinking can make people tired, the feeling comes in an unnatural way, leading to a lower quality of sleep. Between that and the easy waking up, a night of sleep after drinking is hardly restful or helpful to the body. This can lead to extreme tiredness and sluggishness.

Drinking increases the body's temperature through speeding up the heart rate and expanding blood vessels. Though this does make a drinker feel warmer, that heat passes quickly through the skin. This causes the body temperature to fall much faster after it rises. The body also becomes severely dehydrated through introduction to alcohol.

Not every short-term effect is immediately negative; these are some of the reasons people become drawn to drinking. A sense of euphoria and decrease in anxiety can boost some people's perception of themselves or those around them, which is why some people are fun drunks or appear to be. The downside to all of these side effects, however, is that they do not last. Just because someone is less anxious while drinking does not mean their anxiety is cured. A temporary sense of euphoria does not make you the life of the party.

The lowering of inhibitions may be one of the most damaging short-term effects at the moment. While someone is drinking, they are less likely to make sound decisions. They will think that bad decisions are good ones. This is what leads to things like one-night stands, car accidents, or other injuries induced by alcohol. When someone starts dancing on a table or gets behind the wheel after a few drinks, their lowered inhibitions are at work.

When someone is drinking heavily, there is a huge disconnect between the body and the brain. This is what leads to poor decisions, like buying another drink, making bets with a stranger, or getting into a bar fight. The brain becomes pickled due to the alcohol absorbed by the bloodstream. Slower communication, slurred speech, blurred vision, and other side effects weigh heavily on an alcoholic's mind. The real trouble is that those regrets only come after the fact.

In the moment, the drinker realizes almost none of the problems they might be causing. They don't realize they sound or look foolish. A drunk person may not read someone else's body language correctly. This simple problem can lead to numerous issues, especially in a more public place, such as a bar. Someone who is drunk might think that the person sitting beside them is flirting instead of being massively uncomfortable. They may not understand that the bartender is suggesting they slow down. They may not realize that the stranger at the pool table is hustling them.

These recollections and missed signals may be slow in coming to the alcoholic's brain—if they ever do. More than likely, a drunk person will walk away from a night of heavy drinking with no recollection whatsoever. All they will have to show for their night is a headache and an empty wallet in a best-case scenario. Worse scenarios can lead to damage to the car or the body. Arguably, it could be worse still to have bits and pieces of memory rather than a complete blackout.

Imagine this: You've woken up from a night of drinking and your memories are fuzzy. You stumbled to the bathroom, had trouble keeping your balance, but managed to get where you were going. Then, someone grabbed you. Your brain then fails to finish the memory. This leaves you to wonder if you were attacked or if you might have attacked someone when the truth could be simpler. Maybe somebody was just helping you get to a taxi or to your ride home. Even if things were entirely harmless, you may never know for sure because your brain can only provide tiny slivers of memory. The brain is far from the only body part that is affected by alcohol.

Alcohol and Organs

Alcohol circulates through the bloodstream, reaching a wide variety of organs in the body. It starts to break down as soon as it enters your mouth, then goes down your throat and into your digestive system. A small amount of each drink is absorbed by the stomach and small intestine with more alcohol being absorbed by the small intestine if there is no food present in the stomach. If someone drinks after having a meal, the stomach's pyloric sphincter will stay closed to allow the food to be digested. This limits the alcohol's access to the small intestine. Everything that has been absorbed then enters the bloodstream. This provides access to the rest of the body, including important organs such as the brain. Most of what you drink, however, is processed in your liver.

The liver is the largest organ in the human body, sitting just under your ribs on the upper right portion of the abdomen. This organ is responsible for processing nutrients and medicine, storing energy, filtering out toxins, helping blood clot, and making bile to help with the processing of fats—all this in addition to absorbing alcohol. Though there are many factors that can alter this number, the liver can break down, on average, one standard drink per hour. Any additional alcohol consumed in this time will be absorbed by the blood stream, increasing feelings of intoxication.

Most of the alcohol in the liver is processed by an enzyme called alcohol dehydrogenase (ADH), which then turns the alcohol into acetaldehyde. Another enzyme, aldehyde dehydrogenase (ALDH), metabolizes the acetaldehyde into acetate. The acetate is further metabolized to eventually leave the body as carbon dioxide and water. When the blood alcohol level is very high, there is an alternate pathway that activates a different set of enzymes. This is known as the microsomal ethanol-oxidizing system. This system essentially performs the same sort of breakdown, but is equipped to handle larger amounts.

Still, no body of any size or gender can properly process every drop of alcohol that might go into it. This is where the consequences of drinking grow much more serious. Excessive alcohol consumption can cause peptic ulcers in the stomach. It can reduce the pancreas's ability to produce insulin, which can lead to diabetes, or cause the pancreas to become inflamed, leading to pancreatitis. Alcohol is a diuretic, increasing the production of urine. This can change the kidneys' regulation and filtration processes, leading to dehydration.

Alcohol can reach the brain within 30 seconds of consumption. It goes after the nerve cells and the cerebral cortex. This changes the way a person reasons and perceives things, which is why someone who has been drinking only a small amount might think it is a good idea to kiss a stranger or get behind the wheel of a car. Alcohol has a strong effect on memory as well, leading to blackouts, increased aggression, hallucinations, or fatigue.

Drinking too much at once or a large amount over a long period of time can cause an irregular heartbeat, known as arrhythmia. This change in a person's normally steady heartbeat can lead to high blood pressure, as well as severe stretching and/or drooping of the heart muscle, called cardiomyopathy. All of these complications and damage to the heart could result in a stroke, which can be fatal.

Since the liver is in charge of metabolizing the alcohol as it is consumed, this may be the organ that is most affected. Excessive drinking can damage liver cells permanently, turning normal tissue into scar tissue. This alters the liver's ability to absorb nutrients properly, which can lead to an increase in fat accumulation. So much damage also changes the liver's ability to remove toxins from the body. This can result in jaundice, liver failure, or cancer.

According to the National Cancer Institute: "There is a strong scientific consensus that alcohol drinking can cause several types of cancer. In its Report on Carcinogens, the National Toxicology Program of the US Department of Health and Human Services lists consumption of alcoholic beverages as a known human carcinogen.

The evidence indicates that the more alcohol a person drinks—particularly the more alcohol a person drinks regularly over time—the higher his or her risk of developing an alcohol-associated cancer. Even those who have no more than one drink per day and binge drinkers (those who consume four or more drinks for women and five or more drinks for men in one sitting) have a modestly increased risk of some cancers. Based on data from 2009, an estimated 3.5% of cancer deaths in the United States (about 19,500 deaths) were alcohol-related.

Alcohol can cause a number of different cancers. Liver cancer may be the most obvious concern, since that organ is the most responsible for handling alcohol in the body. Excessive drinking can also lead to mouth, throat, esophageal, and laryngeal cancer. All of these, again, are clear concerns since drinking reaches the mouth, throat, and all its component parts first. Chances of developing colon or rectal cancer are increased in heavy drinkers as well. Alcohol has also been linked to prostate cancer, pancreatic cancer, and melanoma.

Alcohol also has a negative effect on the balance of calcium in the body, as well as the production of vitamin D. Both of these are important for bone health. Calcium keeps the bones healthy and vitamin D is one of the things that help the body absorb calcium. Alcoholism can also increase cortisol levels. Cortisol is known to increase the breakdown of bones and decrease the development. Due to all these hormone shifts, falls and broken bones are more common in heavy drinkers, specifically hip or spine fractures.

Alcohol and Calories

The calories in alcohol often get ignored by those who are taking them in. The truth is that calories in alcohol are considered to be empty, meaning they have zero nutritional value. No vitamins, minerals, or anything else necessary to help the body function—just sugar and ethanol. This fact is made even more obvious when checking the nutrition facts on an alcoholic drink. All that is listed is calories, sugar, and carbs. Those extra calories have to go somewhere, which is what connects alcohol and weight gain. But how much are you really taking in?

Wine is usually thought of as a fairly low-calorie alcoholic beverage. The actual calorie count, however, can range from under 100 calories for something like champagne to 160 calories for a sweet or dessert wine. This is per serving. What this means is that a person who has, say, three glasses of wine has taken in the equivalent of half a chocolate cake. A full bottle of wine could add up to the same calorie intake as a multi-patty hamburger.

A pint of beer has between 100 and 150 calories, with some heavier beers, like stout, holding even more calories. This single serving is roughly equivalent to a medium slice of pizza. In other words, someone who drinks a six pack of 16-ounce beers has taken in the same number of calories as are in an entire large pizza.

Mixed drinks can get even higher calorie counts by virtue of the sugary mixers or cola in addition to the alcohol. A frozen margarita has calories similar to a cheeseburger (300 calories on average.) As with all the rest of the drinks discussed here, these calorie counts multiply as more alcohol is ingested. Four standard drinks in one sitting can add up to the same number of calories as two large hot dogs.

All of these numbers are also made very difficult for most people to track or research. Calorie totals are not always made available or easily accessible. They are printed on boxes for multi-packs, but not on individual cans. In bars, the information is rarely available unless a customer asks and a bartender knows where to look. Calorie counts and other facts might not account for changes that can be made to any food or drink order. Just because a single shot of alcohol has only 70 calories does not mean that the count will be the same after soda, more shots, or another type of alcohol is added to the glass. Overall, keeping healthy while drinking is difficult at best.

If you wish to truly keep healthy in the long term, your best bet is to cut back or abstain from drinking. There have been plenty of studies that make a good record of exactly what alcohol does to the human body. Every major organ is affected in some way by virtue of alcohol being absorbed into the blood. The brain and liver are both severely damaged through serious drinking and some of that damage may never heal. Whatever your reasons for wanting to cut back on alcohol, consider your body first and ask yourself what you are really doing to it.

Chapter 2: Types of Alcoholics

"Ignorance is a lot like alcohol: the more you have of it, the less you are able to see its effect on you."—**Jay Bylsma**

The first thing to do, after knowing exactly what alcohol does to your body, is to take a genuinely honest look at your life. Look at your spending, your drinking habits, and the people around you. This last point may be one of the most important. Have any of those around you expressed concern about your drinking? Do they encourage it? Some people believe that a person will emulate the actions and morals of the four people they spend the most time around. This can be something worth considering for those who are trying to cut back on their drinking.

There are many factors that determine how much an alcoholic spends on their habit, including the type of alcohol they drink, where they drink, and the amount they drink. Wine tends to cost more per serving over the long term than beer. Staying constantly buzzed costs more over time than one or two episodes of binge drinking as a person's tolerance goes up. Drinking at a bar costs more than drinking at home. Mixed drinks contain more alcohol and, depending on the drink, can taste less like booze, which makes it harder to track how much alcohol a person is taking in.

Something else to consider is the type of alcoholic you might be; experts in the field of addiction have identified five types: young adults, young antisocial, intermediate familial, functional, and chronic severe. These five types are divided by their age, how much they drink, how likely they are to seek out treatment for their alcoholism, and the treatment that might work best for them, among other factors. Identifying your type may help you to better manage your alcoholism.

The first type of alcoholic is the young adult. This is the most prevalent type in the United States, with 32% of alcoholics falling into the category. Those in the young adult category tend to start drinking at 19 or 20 years old and their average age is around 25. Men in this category are typically single and outnumber women 2.5 to 1.0. They do not commonly have other substance-abuse problems or a history of drinking in the family. These alcoholics drink an average of 143 days in a given year. They favor 12-step programs over private recovery, possibly due to the social aspect.

A young antisocial drinker is also mid-twenties, but they tend to start drinking earlier, generally in the mid-teens. More than half of all young antisocial drinkers have a history of drinking in the family. Their own alcoholic habits emerge within the first two years of beginning to drink. People in this category are also likely to suffer from mental illness. These illnesses can range from antisocial personality disorder to obsessive compulsive disorder to major depression.

Substance abuse is very common with young antisocial alcoholics; many of them abuse opioids, amphetamines, cocaine, or marijuana. Most of them smoke. They tend to drink five or more drinks in a sitting and will drink an average of 200 days in a year. These alcoholics have the most difficult prognosis in terms of possible recovery. Their treatments need to be the most extreme and are more likely to involve a complete cut off from substances rather than cutting back or adding other measures of control.

Functional alcoholics tend to be high-earning and well-educated with good home lives. They are often in denial about their problems with alcohol and tend to make excuses. They tend to start drinking young, at around 18, but do not develop alcoholic habits until their thirties. Though smoking is common for functional alcoholics, they commonly do not have other addictions. One-quarter of functional alcoholics have been diagnosed with depression.

The biggest problem with functional alcoholics is getting them to admit to their problems. Because they do not show obvious signs of severe alcoholism, people in this group are difficult to spot unless you live with them. If they seek help, which only 17% do, these alcoholics will attend 12-step programs or private therapy. Their recovery tends to focus on cutting back to healthy levels or complete abstinence.

Intermediate familial alcoholics start drinking at 17, are middle-aged, and develop alcoholic behaviors in their thirties. Nearly half have a family history of alcoholism. Most have smoked with a quarter of them abusing cocaine and marijuana. Over one-quarter of familial alcoholics have sought help for their addiction. They seek help through their health care providers, self-help groups, detox groups, and other treatment programs.

The final group are the chronic severe alcoholics. Most are middle-aged and started drinking around the age of 16. The vast majority of them smoke and have been diagnosed with co-occurring disorders such as depression, anxiety, or bipolar disorder. These types of alcoholics drink 248 days in a given year. A quarter of people in this category will get divorced. Less than 10% have gone to college and only half are employed full time. Any treatment for chronic severe alcoholics must address their other disorders and include therapies to avoid alcohol relapse.

Drinking Habits

Drinking habits are where, when, and how you drink, among other things. By considering these habits, you can determine which behaviors need to be adjusted in order to allow you to cut back on your drinking. Someone who drinks socially might need to change where they meet with co-workers, skipping the trip to the bar after their shift and heading to a coffee shop instead. A person who drinks at home in the early evening, before dusk, might spend that time away from home with no cash on hand with which to buy alcohol in order to cut back. They might also spend that time with family as a reminder of why they are trying to cut back on drinking. It is important to know your triggers and keep those you can under control.

If you drink when you get stressed, it may be worth investigating alternate means of managing your mood. Meditation or mindfulness could help, as well as reminding yourself that you can only control yourself and your reactions to things. If other people are making you angry, you can choose to let that anger go rather than hide it inside a bottle. Whatever your habits, every person with a drinking problem has them. You probably drink the same type of alcohol at the same time for the same reasons every time. By looking at some of those reasons and triggers, you can successfully cut back. Just be careful to take part in more acceptable behavior while you are trying to cut back.

Drinking on a weekend after all your daily responsibilities are seen to is much more acceptable than catching a drink on your lunch break from work or similar behavior. This kind of irresponsibility could get you hurt or fired or you could hurt someone else. Drinking in the evening is acceptable, but driving to get more booze after you've started drinking is not. If you are engaging in such risky behaviors or if drinking brings out your temper, please consider cutting back, both for your own safety and those around you. These are yet more triggers that can be under your control.

Keep track of how much alcohol you have access to. Perhaps set a daily limit for yourself, especially if you drink at home. Then, make yourself stick to that limit. If necessary, hand your cash or debit card over to whomever you live with and don't reclaim them until your next work shift. For every habit or behavior, there is a work-around if you look hard enough. No matter how much you are drinking now, if you truly wish to cut back, this book can help you do that.

Stages of Alcohol Abuse

Alcohol use disorder is the label used when a person's drinking causes severe distress or harm to their lives. This is common in situations where a person has to drink more than usual to feel the same effects. They may be unable to function without imbibing, which can interfere with daily life. These people may be viewed as selfish due to this inability to put down the booze. This is not true.

Two signs that indicate a physical dependence on alcohol is present include needing to drink more for the same effect. The other sign is suffering withdrawal when alcohol is removed. These symptoms include anxiety, tremors, confusion, nausea, racing heart, and/or sleeplessness. Suffering from withdrawal can further complicate a person's ability to function. All these stages of abuse can lead to some withdrawal symptoms. The level of withdrawal can depend on the level of alcoholism.

The lowest level of alcohol abuse is known as early alcohol abuse. This can be difficult to identify or predict what it may develop into. People at this level will commonly learn about different types of alcohol and are more likely to be experimental drinkers. They will try a wide variety of drinks. They also tend to be social drinkers and will binge drink as a way of partying.

Some people never move past this level of alcohol abuse, drinking only in social situations or during parties. This does not exclude them from the numerous health effects of alcohol use. However, those who do move past this stage to drinking larger amounts more regularly tend to have a history of alcoholism in the family. Other environmental or genetic factors can play a part.

The next level of alcohol abuse is categorized by the amount someone ingests and by the purpose of that ingestion. In other words, those with problematic alcohol abuse will drink with the end goal being drunkenness. These people exhibit physical, emotional, or psychological needs for alcohol. They are more likely to suffer withdrawal symptoms if they are cut off from their source. Any plans for these people to go cold turkey must be medically supervised.

The connection to alcohol and a drinker cannot be ignored at this stage. The need becomes so deeply ingrained that physical withdrawal symptoms are highly likely. Also likely are an increased number of excuses and an increased dependence on drink. These people are less likely to go without regular drinking and are more likely to never walk away from a half-full glass. They are more likely to develop signs of severe alcohol abuse and symptoms of the same.

The third stage is severe alcohol abuse. This is where high-functioning alcoholics are most likely to be found. They will cover up a lot of their drinking or function well enough that others do not suspect. Still, high-functioning alcoholics are not immune to the damage they are doing to their bodies. They can still suffer from anemia, gout, or any of the other diseases that are caused or exacerbated by the presence of alcohol.

End-stage alcohol abuse is the worst stage and those in it have lost most of their hope. They tend to be very self-damaging and are more likely drinking to live rather than living to drink. At this stage, it is less painful to keep reaching for alcohol than to do anything else. Withdrawal would cause extreme pain and organs are commonly failing in these patients. These people are at high risk for intentional self-harm and are often just trying to feel something other than the constant numbing caused by alcohol.

Even in end-stage alcohol abuse, there is still a chance to improve. Though it can be painful, the results are worthwhile. Quitting drinking, or even cutting back, can have amazing effects on a person's health. In some cases, cutting back early enough may help some organs to heal from damage.

No matter what type of alcoholic you are or what therapy you choose, there is always a chance for recovery from addiction if you take the journey seriously. It won't be easy all the time, but it is not impossible either. In fact, if you start with a goal to cut back rather than quit outright, you may be more successful. Knowing the type of alcoholic you are and the stage you might be in can help. Narrowed down options might guide you to the style of therapy and support that is most likely to work for you.

Chapter 3: After the Bar

"Millions of deaths would not have happened if it weren't for the consumption of alcohol. The same can be said about millions of births."—**Mokokoma Mokhonoana**

Drinking has a higher cost to it than just the wallet. This cost can be in the form of lost life, whether through drunk driving accidents, alcohol poisoning, or a bad family environment as a result of drinking. It is often these risks that make people hesitate when it comes to heavy drinking. Alcohol poisoning may be the least problematic of the possibilities because this, at least, is the alcoholic doing something to themselves rather than involving others.

Alcohol poisoning is most often caused by binge drinking, or consuming more than eight to 10 average drinks in a single sitting. Excessive drinking causes 95,000 deaths in the U.S. each year, which averages out to 261 lives lost every single day. Most of these deaths are Caucasian males with an average age of 35. People who die in this way are estimated to shorten their lives by an average of 29 years, according to the Centers for Disease Control (CDC).

Symptoms of alcohol poisoning include slow breathing with less than eight breaths per minute and a gap of 10 seconds or more between breaths. People who have alcohol poisoning can display extreme confusion, nausea, and vomiting. They may have seizures, pass out, or be difficult to wake. Due to alcohol's effect on the body's temperature, someone suffering from alcohol poisoning may also develop clammy skin or even hypothermia. In severe cases, the alcoholic may pass out, slip into a coma, and finally die.

During an alcohol overdose, there is so much alcohol in the blood that the brain begins to shut down basic functions. These include breathing, heart rate, and temperature control. If someone has passed out from drinking, they may choke on their own saliva or vomit and die of asphyxiation. All of this can be made worse through the introduction of drugs or medicines that do not interact well with alcohol. Even if a person does not die from alcohol poisoning, they may suffer brain damage.

Alcohol poisoning and all its associated dangers can be avoided by cutting back on drinking, eating food while drinking to help the body metabolize the alcohol, and not combining alcohol and illegal drugs, among other things. As stated above, though alcohol poisoning is still a loss of life and incredibly tragic, this is, at least, the alcoholic doing something to themselves. When someone gets drunk and makes poor decisions, they may get behind the wheel of a car or go home to an unhappy home and cause even more damage and grief. The effects of drinking too much can touch everyone in an alcoholic's life, some more directly than others. It can even cost a life other than the alcoholic's. Heavy drinking can lead to the deaths of innocent victims.

Drunk Driving

An alcoholic can change the life of a person they have never met in the event of a drunk driving accident. Twenty-eight people die in drunk driving accidents every day. Because alcohol affects the brain, reflexes, and vision, it can severely impair a person's ability to drive safely. Even before reaching levels recognized as drunk, a person who has had alcohol can struggle to perform two tasks at once. Their reduced attention and inability to properly track moving objects only gets worse the more they drink, soon making even the idea of driving all but impossible.

One-third of all traffic fatalities involve a drunk driver. Additionally, up to one-quarter of people feel safe driving after as much as three drinks. After three drinks, still not legally drunk for larger drivers, a person has far less control over their hand-eye coordination, may suffer from short-term memory loss, and might lack ability to properly operate their vehicle, especially in an emergency situation. This has led to 209,000 injuries per year due to impaired drivers.

Drunk driving can cause property damage and legal fees as well. People who get a charge for driving under the influence (DUI) or driving while intoxicated (DWI) are four times more likely to get a second charge or cause loss of life. If someone gets too many charges, they may get a breathalyzer attached to their car. This device is installed for safety in extreme cases and requires the driver to blow a very low BAC number (usually .02 or less) in order to start their vehicle.

These breathalyzers, commonly known as ignition interlock devices, will prevent the vehicle from starting if alcohol is detected in the driver's breath. They commonly consist of a handheld unit, a removable mouthpiece, and a relay cord that hooks into the ignition system. These devices require a very specific pattern of breath strength, pressure, and volume. It is common for a set pattern to be required, such as sucking in, blowing out hard, then sucking in again. These patterns will vary from one device to the next.

These tests are also required at random intervals while the vehicle is being operated. It is suggested that drivers pull over if it is safe to do so in order to conduct these extra breathalyzer tests. If a test is ever failed, the vehicle will not start if it is not already in operation. If it is running, the vehicle may flash the lights, honk the horn, contact the local authorities, or do all of the above. In addition to all of this, the installation of the breathalyzer is usually done at a cost to the vehicle owner.

The other somewhat scary factor to be considered in the question of drunk driving is the presence of any passengers in either vehicle. Half of those polled by the CDC reported that they got in the vehicle with a drunk driver willingly, usually because they were drunk themselves. Most of the time, these people knew the drunk person and trusted that they were okay to drive. This is a common misconception—everyone thinks they are a safer driver than they are, even before alcohol is brought up for consideration. All this behavior does is add to the potential body count in the event of an accident.

No matter how safe a driver you think you are, please remember to be smart about your decisions when it comes to drinking and driving. If you have been drinking, you are statistically far safer getting a ride or using a designated driver to get home rather than getting behind the wheel. This applies even after a single drink. Getting into an accident could cost you property damage, legal fees, or even a life.

Alcohol and the Home

Studies have shown that alcohol abuse and intimate partner violence commonly occur together. The latter can be any type of behavior that causes harm to the partner, including physical, sexual, emotional, or verbal abuse. Alcohol is used as a common excuse in these situations: "I was drunk and upset."

Though not everyone who abuses substances like alcohol or drugs will go on to abuse their partner, there is still a connection there that cannot be denied. Most abusers don't become violent as a result of their substance abuse, but those habits can exacerbate the domestic abuse.

Substance abuse is reported in 40% to 60% of domestic violence cases, according to many studies. This is what suggests the tight connection between the pair of problems. Substance abuse among women who are in a physically abusive relationship are also twice as high when compared to women who are not in an abusive home environment. This can be the woman's own choice, perhaps dulling her pain, or can be done through coercion by her abusive partner. The latter is a common tactic to try and make the victim feel as good, in the moment, as the abuser thinks they feel.

Of course, this does not happen only to women and is not perpetrated only by men. Spousal abuse, just like alcohol abuse, can be practiced by either sex. The addition of alcohol only makes a bad situation worse. If the victim also reaches for alcohol to dull the pain or run away from the problem, you wind up with two alcoholics in the house and nobody has any real self-control or ability to think clearly. It becomes a powder keg.

Many studies have shown that people who take part in domestic abuse will do so after one or more drinks, showing that the level of drunkenness is not a factor. There are also those who abuse their partner without any alcohol entering their system. Alcohol can impact an abuser's perception of a situation, including their reaction to their partner. They might feel more powerful or in control after a drink or two, resulting in a desire for their partner to obey. If their drinking has been a point of argument between them, perhaps due to home finances, drinking can make the fight worse.

Heavy drinking causes a severe erosion of self-control, which can lead to increased aggression or lowered inhibitions. This can cause sexual abuse as well as physical and is commonly reported among college students. Drinking masks shyness and dulls any idea of adherence to rules, leading to increased confidence and loose inhibitions. This increased confidence can be turned up too high as a result of drinking, leading to an expectation of utter obedience from one's partner. A person who feels this way but has no partner may be in an even worse position, expecting obedience from someone who owes them no such thing. This is another situation where domestic violence or sexual abuse is a common result.

These abuses commonly go underreported, either due to improper memory of events or a fear that others may not believe them. This is without considering other possibilities, such as the abuser threatening their victim to remain silent. Another reason for underreporting is a sort of denial about what happened. This is commonly seen in first-time occurrences or younger victims. They may not believe they were actually victimized or be unable to report for fear that others will look on them with pity or disgust.

Alcohol's ability to dull the body and mind have led to it being seriously abused by those who have been hurt in the past, perhaps someone who was physically or sexually abused in childhood. Using alcohol to mask stressors or pain is only effective in the moment and not sustainable over the long term. Eventually, as alcohol tolerance rises, a person will need to drink more to get the same effect. This is why so many who have been abused wind up turning to alcohol to forget their problems. This vicious cycle only leads to more alcohol abuse.

Anyone who may be committing domestic violence as a result of their drinking needs to seek professional help immediately. This is one of the more severe side effects left behind in a life of drinking. Like so many other extreme situations, this can ultimately lead to death of the victim if an abuser does not seek proper help in time. Alcohol and anger are a poor combination and nobody should take that out on their partner. Drinking to fix marital problems is not a fix; it is more akin to sealing a bullet wound with a Band-Aid.

With all of the possible side effects, damages, and other people who can be hurt by a single person's drinking habit, it is incredibly important to look at these habits in full honesty. How much do you drink regularly? How much do you spend on this habit? How do you behave after you have been drinking? How are you treating your partner or other family members? Do you have friends who will be honest with you about your post-drinking behaviors?

A wide variety of strategies can be applied to help someone cut back on their drinking and lessen the secondary effects of this destructive habit. Drinking less and abstaining entirely are two very different strategies, but they can have the same effect in the short term of improving your life. Perhaps choosing to cut back can lead to full abstinence down the line. If the damage you are doing to yourself and others is truly something you wish to decrease or stop, then read on to find strategies that can guide you to drinking less and finding a happier life.

Chapter 4: When, Where, Who, Why

"A full bottle—that was important. Pouring a drink from a half-finished bottle was less comforting than breaking the seal on a fresh one. The comfort lay in knowing you had enough."—**Alex North**, *The Whisper Man*

The drinking habits touched on above are your external obstacles to cutting back or quitting. If you can't ever see yourself giving up alcohol, there is nothing wrong with that, provided you can also keep things under control. If your finances are being drained for the sake of alcohol or you are missing important responsibilities or deadlines because you are drinking too much too often, something needs to change. The first behaviors to examine are those you can change all on your own with little to no outside help.

Drinking in the evenings is generally harmless if all members of your household are accounted for and responsibilities have been completed. This is where the amount of alcohol and the timing may be more significant. If you start drinking at four, as soon as your kids are home from school, you are missing out on bonding time with them and activities like helping them with their homework or playing games. If you are in the habit of buying a large bottle of dark liquor every other day, the amounts you are taking in may be too much.

Evening drinking can be easy to mask if you stay home. Few people put in a real effort toward tracking how much someone else drinks unless they have good reason to do so. Still, there are signs to watch for. Skipping meals or eating smaller amounts may be common for alcoholics. After all, having dinner just lowers the number of calories they can take in from booze. They may eat earlier or stay up later, again, to maximize the time that can be spent drinking.

Day drinkers may function even better than others. After all, drinking during the day means regularly interacting with others. Day drinkers usually look like they have everything more put together, but it's all part of the act. They may not recall who they speak to or what is said. Those who choose to day drink are usually doing something out of the ordinary, even if it is as simple as sitting on a friend's couch rather than their own. From concert venues to sporting events, from hotels to the beach, day drinking is most commonly done away from the home.

An alcoholic will always have money for booze and will make buying it a priority. Most functional alcoholics are not in a position where they will go without paying bills in favor of getting their alcohol, but there are exceptions among heavier drinkers. Even if money is tight, an alcoholic will find a way to purchase whatever they can afford. Most would rather buy a single 24-ounce can of beer than go without.

One of the best ways to analyze your drinking habits and how big a problem they might be is to consider how well you wake up in the mornings. How many days in a given week are you hungover? How often do you reach for the "hair of the dog" upon waking up? It is common for someone hungover to sample some of the same drink from the previous night, believing it will lessen the severity of hangover symptoms. The truth is, this practice only gets you closer to getting drunk again. It offers no recovery time and makes hangovers worse.

Drinking at home may be safer, relatively speaking, and tends to be the preferred location of some alcoholics. After all, drinking at home means there is less risk of driving. It also lessens the chances that an alcoholic will be cut off. You are more likely to run out of alcohol at home than stop yourself from drinking or have someone else suggest you stop. In fact, this is often the only thing that can even slow down a homebound alcoholic once they have started drinking.

Drinking in a bar can offer a more social atmosphere since there are generally more people around. Some bars even provide activities for their patrons, like pool tables or special karaoke nights. The greater risks here do involve other people. Misunderstandings can lead to bar fights, drinks can be contaminated, and everyone still has to make it home at the end of the night. A bar can offer a sense of acceptance, allowing an alcoholic to become a familiar face among like-minded people. Still, depending on the others in the bar, you may wind up unsupported or shunned if you share your plans to cut back.

Drinking Partners

Social drinking is a common practice in America. Where there are adults, there will likely be alcohol if it is appropriate to the environment. Co-workers meet at bars after work, people drink at parties or festivals, and alcohol does seem to make an appearance wherever there might be a crowd. Alcohol, in fact, is a common social lubricant, used to help people relax and talk to one another. Events such as bar trivia form a link between drinking and competitiveness, as do party games like beer pong.

A group of adults getting together to have a few drinks and chat is a positively ancient idea, often practiced by Greek philosophers. Studies show that people experience lowered inhibitions, less anxiety, and have more energy while drinking. This makes it a natural choice of beverage to loosen tongues and get conversation going. Social drinking doesn't even require a large group. Even a first date falls under the category of social drinking.

The idea of drinking socially is not a problem on its own. As with all other things, it is a question of numbers and moderation. In fact, a social drinker is defined as someone who only drinks a few times a month, no more than once a week, and has no more than three standard drinks in that time. Meeting for one or two drinks with a coworker is generally harmless. Likewise, few people would look twice if someone got a couple of drinks while on vacation. This only becomes problematic when heavy drinking or binge drinking behaviors emerge.

The trouble with moderating alcohol intake if a person never drinks on their own is the addition of peer pressure. After all, as many people might point out, one drink never hurts anything. This is also why social drinking can lead to heavier habits. If someone always reaches for a drink when one is offered to them, they can lose track of how much they've taken in. This sort of behavior can lead to more dangerous situations, such as alcohol poisoning or date rape situations.

Even without those extremes, the act of social drinking may lead to worse habits. After all, your friends could be learning, inadvertently, that you only spend time with them when alcohol is provided. Therefore, they may make it a point to make sure it is there before they invite you. There may also be members of the group who are alcoholics themselves and are not yet ready to face the truth about their addiction. Either of these scenarios can make things very difficult for someone who is looking to cut back.

It is important to be honest with those you spend regular time with, especially if they join you or encourage social drinking. If you want to cut back, set firm limits and stick to them. You may decide to reward yourself with one drink at a social event following several days of sobriety. Stick with that promise to yourself. If your friends decide not to listen, be firm with them. Proper phrasing, safe ways to refuse drinks, and sticking to boundaries will be addressed more in depth in a later chapter.

If your friends or family still refuse to listen and try to ply you with more alcohol during social situations, you need to find alternatives. You may need to distance yourself from some people who are important to you. You'll need to decide if this is a break you want to make quickly and cleanly or if you'd rather explain and give them a chance to understand and accept your new limitations. More drastic choices may be needed to help you cut back on your drinking.

If you drink around coworkers, the solution may be as easy as suggesting a new place to meet. Festivals or parties can be enjoyed with non-alcoholic beverages, which are almost always an option at any location. Restaurants and bars, in particular, are fully capable of catering to those who choose not to imbibe. Practicing in social situations without alcohol can lessen the need for it as a social lubricant. Try chatting first with those you are more comfortable with and just allow conversation to flow naturally. There is no need to fill every pause or beat of quiet. With time, you may find out you are a fine conversationalist without any alcohol in your system.

For those who have cut back or quit alcohol altogether, social drinking might be a way to reintroduce the idea and test your own tolerance. It may be possible to enjoy these kinds of safe drinking behaviors as a way to still enjoy alcohol without losing control entirely. Just be careful and be honest with yourself if destructive behaviors begin to emerge again. Some heavy drinking alcoholics may need to completely abstain and there is nothing wrong with that. Every person is different. What matters is that you have support around you as you try to abstain or cut back. The easiest place to start looking for this group is among those with whom you normally drink.

Reasons to Drink

There are many reasons that people might decide to drink. Peer pressure is a big factor. Whether a person is celebrating their 21st or attending a party for a friend, the number of people around seems to directly increase the odds that alcohol will be present and be offered. Many people start drinking simply to fit in or to avoid looking silly. This is because of alcohol's previously mentioned abilities as a social lubricant. With everyone else drinking and having a good time, somebody who might not be inclined to drink might worry about bringing the party down and wind up drinking instead.

Social anxiety adds to peer pressure as the desire to fit in might make a person feel more worried or anxious the longer that they do not appear to fit in. There is a commonality between alcoholics and people with social anxiety disorder. In fact, those who suffer from social anxiety are 20% more likely to develop a drinking problem. This usually happens 10 years after the anxiety disorder diagnosis.

Stress can be another external factor. Since alcohol dulls the nervous system, it can numb many emotions as well. A stressed-out person might relax emotionally, mentally, and physically after having a few drinks. People who are drinking tend to forget things and this might include details around different stressors. After all, you can't stress out over something you've forgotten.

Some people drink just to feel good. The euphoria and joy of many drinks is enough of a draw to have a person happy to be the life of the party. There are many who develop their whole personality or a public persona around this idea. Most crazy partiers don't let others see what happens when the party ends. In fact, those who reach for alcohol to feel good are more likely to suffer from depression and will drink to mask those feelings.

Depression is another common reason to drink. The previously mentioned numbing and euphoria can combine to offer a reprieve from depression. Because this is not a common feeling, people are more likely to independently seek it out for themselves. We drink to feel good.

There are those for whom drinking may be a learned behavior. Some people grow up exposed to alcohol and alcoholics, making them more likely to drink themselves. Since alcohol was always around, these people may downplay the side effects and damage many alcoholics experience. Some may even be fortunate enough to show fewer signs of this damage and think it does not apply to them.

Addictive personality types are also likely to be drinkers. These people may start drinking due to peer pressure or early exposure or any of the above reasons. They will keep going because they cannot stop. An addictive personality is more inclined to need external stimulation and then will be drawn to the results of said stimulation. Alcohol, illegal drugs, and other high-risk behaviors are all natural draws for addictive personalities.

Some people just like the taste of specific drinks, but this is highly subjective and not a primary reason a person might turn to abusing alcohol. There are as many reasons to drink as there are people who drink. Very few alcoholics, however, turn to drinking as a regular habit because things are going well for them. Usually, there is some trauma or pressure helping to draw someone slowly into alcoholism. Recognizing what the cause of your own alcohol abuse might be can help you to have an easier time in cutting back.

Chapter 5: Setting Boundaries

"Meanwhile the 3 a.m. drunks of the world would lay in their beds, trying in vain to sleep, and deserving that rest, if they could find it."—**Charles Bukowski**

One of the most difficult decisions you can make is to cut back your alcohol intake. You are agreeing to give up or, at least, lessen a lot of the enjoyment you may derive from drinking. You are interrupting some long-held habits and will need to replace them with something. If you don't find some suitable replacement, you may return to alcohol simply because it is available. First, however, before any of that, you need to set boundaries with yourself and the people around you.

Setting these with yourself may be easier and might include things like limiting the amount of cash you carry to buy drinks with. If that safeguard is not enough, you could leave your credit or debit card at home. Perhaps you will limit yourself to a six pack per day in your efforts to cut back. Maybe you will change the route you take to get home to keep from driving past the liquor store or local bar.

If you are an at home drinker, you might seek out activities after work to keep yourself busy during a portion of the time you would normally spend drinking. If you are away from home and the familiar triggers of getting off work and walking in the door or having dinner with family are not there, your brain cannot automatically go to the next expected behavior. This can also expose you to new people, places, and things. Maybe you will do a picnic dinner once a week with family or similar.

The other big difficulty involves other people. As many people claim, the hardest part is admitting you have a problem. Oftentimes, when someone speaks to their friends or family about their own alcohol addiction, their honesty is met with denial. "You're not that bad. You don't drink that much. You've never caused problems. You function just fine!" These reactions are common for many reasons.

First, the family and friends of alcohol abusers often do not see the signs and symptoms unless they are living with the alcoholic. Some functional alcoholics manage to hide their struggles and symptoms for years and are still greeted with disbelief. This is part of the nature of the disorder as well as how acceptable alcohol is considered by society. People don't commonly consider drinking to be a problem if the person taking the drinks isn't being dangerous. No drunk driving? No problem. No violence? You're fine.

Second, there are many who will excuse alcohol under most circumstances. Everyone drinks. It is such a socially acceptable habit that many people who are not living with serious addicts will think nothing of someone choosing to drink alcohol. On the other hand, those who have lived with addicts are more likely to develop a zero-tolerance policy for the sake of their loved one. Some alcoholics are able to simply cut back on their drinking. Others have to abstain entirely. Friends and family tend to follow the lead of the addict they know.

No matter the excuses or struggles, many alcoholics have to be honest about their addiction and handle it. The care and support of loved ones can help, of course, but alcoholics must set their own limits to cut back on their drinking. This is why setting boundaries is very important. The challenge here can be telling those around you that you are cutting back on drinking. You need to plan carefully what you might say and be ready to be very firm with those in your life. Being firm may be the most important point, in fact.

Many people are not used to setting or listening to boundaries. People just plain don't like boundaries if their behavior is being affected. Ironically, the same sort of people who might declare your boundaries ridiculous or silly would also expect their boundaries to be treated as nearly holy. This double standard is painfully common among those who think their limits should be important to everyone around them. These same people might ignore your boundaries entirely.

You must know your limits, what you will tolerate, and what you won't. Communicate these boundaries clearly, maybe giving a warning to those who might be pushing at your limits. "Hey, I told you I'm not going to drink. Please don't ask again." After one or two warnings, do not be afraid to walk away entirely and tell them this will happen. "Listen, I've told you I'm not going to do that. If you ask again, I'm leaving." Following such a warning, you must stand by what you say. Carry out whatever consequences you promised.

When to Set Boundaries

Setting boundaries can be difficult if people don't respect them. The first thing you need to know as you decide what boundaries to set is what rights you have. These rights can help you to know when your boundaries are being overstepped. They may not be what many would think of in regards to boundaries; these rights are things like the right to say no without feeling guilty or the right to make your needs as important as everyone else's. In other words, these rights are the very things that people tend to struggle with when they decide to set boundaries.

Boundaries are often ignored, either by the person who set them or by those around them when these rights are also disregarded. Everyone also has their own reasons for trying to ignore other people's boundaries. "You helped me out last time." "It's just this once." "You did it for someone else." "I really need it." In some cases, these may not be reasons as much as excuses and you are likely to know.

It is important to listen to your body when you are setting and sharing the details of your boundaries with others. Your instincts and your body's automatic reactions will tell you when someone is pushing too far and a boundary is either needed or being violated. If you tense up every time a certain person offers their unsolicited opinion, you need to have some sort of boundary with that person. Maybe they need to understand that the more opinions they offer, the less likely you are to listen.

Boundaries are shaped by our heritage, culture, personal morals, life experiences, and how we interact with others. Knowing when, how, and with whom to set up a healthy boundary is key. People who exhaust you or wear you out might need some boundaries to put them at some distance from you. Remember, you are not setting these boundaries to be mean. You are doing it for your own mental and physical health.

When setting boundaries around alcohol, you may need to do more than just say you are quitting drinking. You might need to spend less time around former drinking buddies or distance yourself from people who cause you unnecessary stress. It can also help to find other locations to spend your leisure time. Instead of the bar, go to a park or restaurant. If you attend a party, request a non-alcoholic drink up front and do not apologize for that need. Keep your boundaries firm, whether they are with others or with yourself.

Setting boundaries with others can be difficult because people don't always listen. Likewise, it can be a challenge to set boundaries for yourself for the same reason. As the joke goes, "I gave myself a deadline, but I know who did that and he's an idiot." Some of the time, we are even less likely to listen to ourselves than we are to listen to others. The boundaries we can set for ourselves also revolve around things like self-control, for which we can easily make our own excuses.

Healthy boundaries, no matter who they involve, are those that allow us room to grow and be vulnerable. If you are oversharing about your troubles with alcohol, for example, and telling everyone you come across, you may need to set a boundary. Likewise, if you are not sharing anything and hiding your bad habits, you might adjust that boundary to allow a select few people in. Boundaries are not meant to be unscalable walls that nobody can cross, nor are they lines in the sand for a person to step right over.

Accepting the word 'no' is another sign of a healthy boundary and this goes both ways. You are allowed to say no without any guilt and so is the person or people you are speaking with. Nobody has to agree to do anything that makes them uncomfortable. A refusal to do something should never lead to a guilt trip and does not require an explanation.

Healthy boundaries are designed not to exclude people for no reason. If there is a person you may need to spend less time with while you try to quit drinking, it will be for a reason. Maybe they offer you alcohol when they shouldn't. Maybe they drink more than you are comfortable with. Nobody will get cut from your life as a result of a boundary for any kind of made-up reason. Anyone who might think that can ask for more information on what and why you have the boundaries you do. You still don't owe them an answer unless you want to give it.

How to Stick to Your Boundaries

When setting boundaries, it is important to be assertive without being aggressive. This allows the boundaries to feel firm to others without people getting mad or feeling like they are being attacked. One important way to do this is by using "I statements." These serve to make specific boundaries nonnegotiable without placing blame or using threats. One example of an I statement could be "when we go to the bar and I'm not drinking, I feel left out because I can't buy any alcohol. What I need is for us to go somewhere that doesn't serve alcohol once or twice a week." The boundary, a reason for it, and an alternative are all mentioned without making anyone involved feel bad about the situation.

I statements are designed to express thoughts, feelings, and opinions without needing to consider the same of others. This is important because your boundaries apply to you and nobody else. I statements are also a good form of effective communication. Simply getting upset and venting your feelings about a situation is not helpful in the long run. "I don't want to go to the bar anymore" is an accurate statement, but not a helpful one.

Learning to say no is another important thing to practice when keeping to boundaries. Remember that no is a complete sentence all on its own. Some people are hesitant to say no without any further explanation or details, but that is not required at all. You owe nobody an explanation for the boundaries you set or why you need to set them.

Setting boundaries for your belongings, physical space, and your time can also be very important and helpful when trying to cut back on alcohol. For example, if you are buying a six pack for yourself and limiting yourself only to those six beers, it is perfectly acceptable to have those beers be only there for you to drink. You aren't required to share with anyone or to explain why you are not doing so. Setting boundaries on your time can also be effective. Maybe you agree to go to the bar, but only for 30 minutes and only spending a set amount of money on yourself. If you are not buying rounds for friends or accepting free drinks from them, you can control how much you take in.

Other boundaries you can set when trying to quit drinking may include things like not having alcohol in your home aside from what you purchase. You might decide that casual discussion of booze is not allowed. People who live with you may be banned or encouraged, depending on what you want to do, to ask how much you have been drinking. Encouraging this can serve as a way to keep you honest as well as accountable to others.

Though creating boundaries is not always a popular thing, it is very important for anyone who wishes to see their goals actually succeed. Without boundaries, you could find yourself being dragged to bars or buying alcohol as if you had never expressed any wish to cut back. This is no good at all. Being firm about boundaries is just as important as setting them. You also need to set boundaries for yourself as well as those around you. Just make sure they are not unreasonable.

An important factor in setting reasonable boundaries is allowing yourself and those around you a little bit of grace. You will not be able to walk away from alcohol with no warning or cutting back. Likewise, friends who are used to drinking with you regularly may need gentle reminders before they stop inviting you to the bar on a daily basis. Family members who are used to getting beers for you may habitually go to the fridge. These things will happen. It is all a force of habit. When these habitual slips do happen, you should not blame yourself or those who are trying to help you.

At the same time, you need to be honest with yourself. There are some alcoholics who say they are trying to cut back, but give excuses rather than boundaries. "It was a hard day at work." "I'm anxious and need to unwind." "I'll never survive this party without a beer or two." "There was only one left in the case." If you are giving these sorts of excuses and accepting them from yourself, try rephrasing them as I statements to learn what your true motivation might be.

"Work was tense and I want to relax with a drink because...." "There was just one left in the case and I need it now because...." Many of these excuses, then repurposed as I statements, do not have very good endings. Not the sort of thing you would want to repeat to someone else if they asked for further details.

Make sure you are setting boundaries that align with your goals. Do not set redundant boundaries or any that will not truly help you. Your boundaries, much like your goals, need to be specific, measurable, attainable, reasonable, and time oriented. "I won't drink more than a six pack tomorrow night." This boundary is specific to the next night, measurable by virtue of the number of drinks you are limiting yourself to, and is something you can absolutely succeed at with just a little self-discipline.

When setting goals and boundaries, make sure you are surrounding yourself with people who will support you. You may have friends or family members who will be pleased to hear about your efforts to cut back on drinking and excited to hear any updates you can give along the way. It is also possible that there are people in your life who have struggled with their own drinking habits. In this case, there is a built-in support network for you to draw on when you need it. Make sure those you surround yourself with will support your goals of trying to drink less. You never know when one extra word of kindness or a supportive ear might make all the difference.

Chapter 6: Regulate and Replace

"Alcohol is the only drug in the world where, when you stop taking it, you are seen as having a disease."—**Holly Whitaker**, *Quit Like a Woman: The Radical Choice to Not Drink in a Culture Obsessed with Alcohol*

Once you have set a goal to cut back on your alcohol intake, it may be best to start as soon as possible. Drinking less will mean you are taking in fewer calories, which can lead to better health. You will also need to replace the caloric intake that used to account for your drinking. This is where you can make some smarter choices: water, juice, healthier drinks, and less greasy food. Juice, specifically, should be seriously considered as part of your goal in cutting back on alcohol.

The question of replacing calories can be a tricky one, especially when cutting out alcohol can lead to sugar cravings. The reason for these cravings is that sugar, like alcohol, triggers the release of dopamine and serotonin in the brain. These feel-good chemicals are part of what causes alcohol to be so addictive. This replacement of one substance for another for the sake of creating specific brain chemicals is known as addiction transfer. However, when it comes to alcohol and sugar replacement, this is only the beginning of possible problems.

Over 95% of former drinkers develop hypoglycemia or low blood sugar. Glucose, a simple sugar in your blood, serves as fuel for your brain, so when it is low, you can't function well. Cutting down on alcohol cuts down on the glucose your body can draw from. This can lead to irritability, confusion, and anxiety.

Craving sugar while trying to cut back or quit alcohol is normal and not something you should try to ignore. Your body is struggling to maintain the blood sugar level it is used to and your brain is lacking in feel-good chemicals, both as a result of the lower amounts of alcohol you are taking in. This is not a question of willpower, but of the body crying out for what it needs. So, don't fight it. If you need some extra snacks or desserts for a few evenings instead of reaching for alcohol, it's okay.

Some people do still feel guilty about reaching for sugar as a replacement for an alcohol addiction. There are many ways to ease these sugar cravings, including eating at regular intervals. In the early days of sobriety, skipping meals or waiting too long to eat can increase your cravings as your body's need for calories goes up. You need to plan on eating something every four hours or so with snacks in between traditional mealtimes. Focus on fat, protein, and fiber rather than just carbs. All that carbs will do is convert to simple sugar, which puts you in the same position you were already in.

Protein is important, especially at breakfast, which tends to be a carbohydrate heavy meal. Carbs, just like sugar, will lead to energy crashes as your body depletes its fuel stores faster. So, add peanut butter to your toast or cook an extra egg. Protein, healthy fat, and fiber will keep your blood sugar levels in balance. These nutrients will also give your body the raw materials it needs to begin recovery from your drinking. High-protein snacks can also be helpful in the middle of the day, when energy levels naturally drop.

While you are considering what kind of food you take in, the amounts and timing, and how much alcohol you are looking to replace, it is important to plan for this energy drop. Alcohol and complex carbohydrates both tend to be easy items to grab when a craving hits and are very effective at chasing them off, but can only lead to more of the troubles you are currently having. Better to go for fresh fruit. Hard-boiled eggs or nuts make for another easy grab-and-go snack.

If you struggle with or are unable to replace the full number of calories you are taking in through alcohol, there are other steps you can take to change the amount you are taking in. Buying less alcohol is an obvious solution, but many people struggle with the idea. The whole idea of regulating alcohol intake is commonly mocked or belittled, especially among men. There is an idea that men are allowed to reach for a beer to escape whatever their troubles may be. This is so accepted that some guys get teased when they announce any intention to quit. Even if you decide not to make your cutting back a public decision, there are still steps you can take to cut back on calories, sugar, and alcohol content.

You can buy smaller amounts of alcohol to regulate how much you can drink. Switching to a light beer or similar lighter form of alcohol can also change the number of total calories you are ingesting. Get food anytime you drink and do not be afraid to add a glass or pitcher of water to keep yourself hydrated as you imbibe. All of these small changes require a new level of awareness, a little bit of extra care.

If you are buying your own alcohol at a grocery store or similar as opposed to a bar, track the percentage of alcohol in your drink as well as the calories. Something that is 20% alcohol by volume (ABV) contains more than a drink that is 8% ABV. This measurement tells how much alcohol is in the entire container. So a 15-ounce can at 3% ABV is 45% alcohol.

At some bars, you may be able to ask for a lighter drink that doesn't contain large amounts of alcohol. Light beers, white wines, and singles over doubles in mixed drinks are some of the ways to limit your alcohol intake. Smaller portions and smaller containers are also fantastic methods to cut back on how much you drink. These may be easier steps to take than working the math each time.

It is also important not to let yourself be tempted by sales or specials. Do not buy a larger amount of alcohol because of a sale. If six packs are buy one get one half off, but you only planned to buy one, stick with that plan. Spending more money is rarely the deal people make it out to be, no matter what you are buying. After all, you are purchasing more than you originally planned.

Any time you are at a bar or restaurant, you will need to stay aware of the wait staff or bartenders around you. Otherwise, an over-eager employee may pour more than you want to drink. This will not be deliberate on their part, but could land you in the same position regardless of their intentions. Too many people drink too fast, even though small fill-ups over time still add to their body's BAC.

This idea of practicing awareness is exactly why you need to know the limits you are setting for yourself. After all, if you do not know where the finish line is, how will you know when you've crossed it? In other words, without hard limits set ahead of time, how will you know when to stop? Setting these limits can be hard because some people want to push. This is part of setting firm boundaries with yourself and others.

A common suggestion for those in this position is keeping no alcohol whatsoever in the home. This is where support from friends and family can be irreplaceable. If those closest to you know you are trying to cut back, they might be willing to help by following the boundaries you set. You could, for example, choose only to buy alcohol in specific amounts on specific days of the week as opposed to every evening. If you have to keep drinks in your home, these limits are inescapably important. One six pack, three nights a week might be reasonable, but it must be maintained.

Keeping no alcohol in the home, on the other hand, can limit the amount of temptation someone is exposed to while trying to cut back. A temptation is much harder to ignore when it is physical. In other words, wanting to go out and get more alcohol is a desire that can be ignored or buried. However, if it's just in the next room, waiting and cold, refusal becomes much more difficult.

Setting specific goals for yourself can help you to celebrate more when you have met them. This allows a better appreciation of any struggles you faced while trying to meet the goal. You just need to remember that a goal is not a be all, end all deadline. If your goal is not met at first, adjust accordingly.

A goal to drink just a six pack a day might be too much, depending on your normal intake. It could be more attainable to say "I have been drinking 10–12 drinks a night. I'm going to cut down to eight drinks per night over the next week." This is still cutting down, though not so much to make the effort unbearable. If you do not succeed the first week, that doesn't mean you are doomed to failure. Just re-examine the goal and adjust. Maybe instead of every night, you can try for every other night. The other important factor in such adjustable goals is not to use attainability as an excuse to binge. Dropping your intake three nights a week does not mean you binge extra drinks outside of those nights to make up for what you missed. The goal, after all, is to cut back. You do yourself no good in the long run if you cut back to six packs during the week, only to buy 30 packs on the weekends.

Alcohol Withdrawal

While you are trying to cut back on your drinking, it is a good idea to log your efforts. This will allow for posterity as well by providing a written account so that you can see yourself improving over time. You can track in a journal or on a computer spreadsheet. You can even jot quick notes in your cell phone. Things to keep track of include how much you are drinking, the type of alcohol, when and where you are drinking it, and your mood. You may also want to keep any symptoms written down.

The symptoms of cutting back on alcohol, much like those symptoms caused by heavy drinking, can be physical, mental, or emotional. Symptoms can also be experienced either by those who are cutting back on their drinking or those who are abstaining completely. People who intend to quit drinking completely tend to experience more severe symptoms, but that does not mean that others are exempt. Some symptoms of alcohol withdrawal can start to show up just a few hours after the last drink. These start as mere hangover symptoms, but they can become worse depending on how much the person had to drink.

Because alcohol slows the brain, more chemicals are released to compensate for the drink's depressive effects. These extra chemicals are then overproduced compared to those who do not drink. As this becomes the brain's new normal, that production of extra chemicals does not stop just because the alcohol is present in lower amounts. The extra chemicals are still there and can send the alcoholic into a state of overstimulation. This does not last more than a few days, but can still be unpleasant.

Irritation, fatigue, and feelings of jumpiness or nervousness are a few signs of alcohol withdrawal. These, however, could also be attributed to a bad hangover. The presence of extra stimulating chemicals can cause noises to seem too loud, lights too bright. Combined with difficulty thinking clearly, the assault on the senses pairs with a scrambled mind and leads to severe mood swings. The fatigue, anxiety, and random bursts of energy are all a result of the simple sugars absent in the blood. Because these sugars may be a regular source of fuel for the body, limiting them can lead to physical symptoms as well

Clammy skin, elevated blood pressure, and headaches are only the start of what's to come as the body processes the last dregs of alcohol and no more is forthcoming. Sweating, hand tremors, and paleness are easy identifiers for someone in the grip of withdrawal. Insomnia and vomiting are two symptoms that may commonly keep people from cutting back. They would rather deal with hangovers and risk their body than go through withdrawal. The symptoms of withdrawal are a common reason for relapses as well. People will reach for a drink to make their withdrawal symptoms stop. This starts the entire cycle over again.

There is another, more severe form of withdrawal usually only seen in very severe alcoholics. This is known as delirium tremens, and those who suffer from it are often malnourished prior to the symptoms setting in. Roughly one in every 20 people who develop delirium tremens will die as a result. This extreme form of alcohol withdrawal requires medical attention until the symptoms have subsided. Fever, hallucinations, tremors, and seizures are some common signs that someone is experiencing delirium tremens.

Though severe symptoms can last longer, as in the case of delirium tremens, there is also an accepted timeline of common withdrawal symptoms. Things can start anywhere between four and 12 hours of a person's last drink. These symptoms are also experienced by anyone who has developed a dependence on alcohol, whether they are cutting back their drinking or quitting altogether. The primary difference is the severity of symptoms people experience.

Acute alcohol withdrawal tends to be at its worst two days after quitting with symptoms improving around day five. These are restlessness, insomnia, irritability, mood swings, and trouble eating. Some mild symptoms, such as anxiety or insomnia, can remain present at a lower intensity for up to six months. Severe symptoms, such as hand tremors, fainting, or sweating, could lead to delirium tremens. Delirium tremens can appear in the first four days of quitting drinking, but may also take up to 10 days to manifest. These severe symptoms can last up to five days.

These withdrawal symptoms can be uncomfortable, to say the least, and have an effect on everyone who lives close to the alcoholic going through them. It is a struggle for all involved, but is still only temporary in the long run. Don't let a few days of discomfort prevent you from doing what you need to do for yourself and those you care about. Staying hydrated, keeping sugar levels up, and affording yourself the grace of forgiveness are all ways to lessen withdrawal symptoms or make things easier in general. You can get through withdrawal successfully and make it to the other side where you can look at recovery options.

Why Regulate and Replace Matters

Whether you are drinking a 30 pack every weekend or a 12 pack each night, your decision to cut back on drinking probably means that the drink has more control over your life than you want. When this is the case, just saying you want to cut back is not enough. You need to change how much you are imbibing in order to actually cut back. Putting in this effort will help you to feel better about yourself and your decision. Drinking less will also provide you with income no longer spent on alcohol. These extra savings can add up very fast over time.

Regulating how much you drink not only provides proof of progress, but ensures that you stay in control of your habits. You making the choice for yourself of how much you can drink returns a small portion of power to you. Setting these limits on yourself is about more than cutting back. It proves you still have a hand on the metaphorical wheel. You make the decisions for yourself.

Careful regulation of alcohol intake can also change how and when withdrawal symptoms hit as well as how severe they are. If you cut back with a methodical approach and take your time with it, you raise your odds of success. Your tolerance can't rebuild if your intake doesn't do the same. Because of this, your overall health will improve and your body can begin to heal. If, on the other hand, you fall back on old habits, you do yourself no favors and can even make things worse than they were before. When someone cuts back and then returns to drinking too quickly, they will return to their previous levels with little difficulty. This can lead to getting drunk faster and staying that way longer.

Replacing habitual behaviors like drinking and any habits or routines tied to it is another step to ensure your success. Rather than go to the bar and find a non-alcoholic drink, you might suggest a change of venue to reduce your own temptation. You can use excuses if others are pressuring you to drink. An early work day, medication that interacts poorly with alcohol, or being a designated driver are all excuses that do not afford many questions or objections. You can also volunteer to be the designated driver rather than just use it as an excuse. This will allow you to spend time with your friends and know that everyone riding with you makes it home safe regardless of how much they drank.

This gaining of different habits and behaviors is intended to break the cycles you might have established. Meeting somewhere other than the bar can distance you from temptation. Carrying less cash and no cards or checks will limit how much alcohol you can buy. Designated driving can eliminate the problem altogether for the nights you choose to take that route. If your usual friend group drinks all the time, maybe you can spend some time with family instead. Your partner or kids will probably love spending time with you. Seeing you fully sober, interacting freely, can also offer a glimpse of the goal you are working toward and the future you might all have together.

Changing habits and behaviors might include some unusual ones, like paying for fuel at the pump instead of going inside. You might buy soda where you once bought beer, thereby replacing the sugars as well as the psychological need for a cold drink. If your alcohol of choice always goes into a specific glass in your home, you might consider getting rid of that glass. Similarly, if your alcoholic drinks always contain ice or a straw, you might abandon those briefly to keep your mind from expecting alcohol where there is none. If you want the flavor of a mixed drink without the alcohol content, you could try things like buying alcohol free mixers and drinking them plain.

You might want new ways to fill time once dedicated to drinking. If you like watching competitive sports, leaving to get drinks will make you miss something, whether you are watching live or televised. Taking part in sports or exercise can add a feeling of competition and fun to your life that might be able to replace some of the joy you used to get from opening a drink. Exercising or competitive sports can also increase your overall health. Going outdoors, weather permitting, will give you more fresh air and sunshine. This, again, can improve your overall health.

You can use this time to improve yourself in a variety of ways. Maybe you want to learn a new skill. Playing an instrument, building a shelf, writing a book—there is a wide variety of possibilities out there. If you wish to fill time formerly spent drinking, it will be better in the long run to seek some new skill or experience. You could make a new craft or learn to dance. Some of these ideas can also help you to meet new people and spend time at places other than the local bar, thereby keeping you from your normal habits and temptation.

No matter what you choose to fill your time or replace your drinking, there are sure to be benefits to be gained. Cutting back on drinking and making new friends or learning a new skill at the same time is a great thing. By determining what behaviors and hobbies you want to have other than drinking, you can find a new friend group or perhaps be reintroduced to your old one. Most people behave differently while drinking. If you can encourage your friends to join you in a non-drinking activity, you can reconnect with them as people, away from the booze. This can strengthen friendships and help you to know who might still be with you after you've become less of a drinker.

New habits and strict restrictions around your drinking habits will make it easier to cut back. Find new environments and new people to spend time with, if you wish. Going to places where alcohol isn't allowed may give you a greater appreciation for entertainment venues you had never considered before. You should not hesitate to fill time that would ordinarily be used for drinking, doing whatever you can to prevent old habits from taking over. You can learn new card games or kindle an old love for reading. The sky's the limit! This searching for different hobbies can reveal new talents, new skills, and new friends. In time, it may reveal a new you as well.

Chapter 7: Seeking Help

"When you are young, you drink to be sociable, and when you are old, you drink to be unsociable."—**Robert Black**

A recovering alcoholic can seek a variety of ways to get help. After all, most of us cannot go it alone where serious addiction is concerned. There is nothing wrong with asking for help, but what help do you ask for in this situation? The first thing many people do is consult their doctors. This makes sense, considering the effect alcohol has on the body. When speaking with your doctor, just like when you first analyzed your behaviors for yourself, you need to be honest. Don't sensationalize, but don't lie either. If you are regularly imbibing 10 standard drinks every night, just tell your doctor that.

Your doctor is likely to ask several questions about your drinking habits and may ask to speak to family or friends for a more complete picture of the situation you are in. However, this will not happen without your permission, and those the doctor speaks with will not be given private information about you. A physical exam will happen so that you can be checked for any damage that might be caused by your drinking. Lab tests and imaging orders are also common. These will involve x-rays or ultrasounds and blood draws. They are to further check for damage.

There are no specific tests for alcohol use disorder, but some commonalities in symptoms can point to it. These include things like liver damage, abnormal blood sugar levels, and abnormal blood pressure among other things. All of these signs are a side effect of alcohol working on the body as discussed in Chapter 1. These symptoms, much like organ damage, do not disappear easily. They will be there for your doctor to see for up to a week after a period of serious drinking, depending on what signs the doctor may be looking for.

A variety of medical intervention steps can be explored to help people who want to cut back on their drinking. An inpatient stay will most likely happen in severe cases where the person's drinking makes them an obvious danger to themselves or others. This commonly involves the patient being held in the hospital while they detox from their drinking. Detoxification is a special word for a medically supervised withdrawal. Sedating medicines can be given in order to lessen the withdrawal symptoms.

Psychological counseling commonly happens for inpatient as well as outpatient treatment. This can involve steps such as facing the reality of one's drinking and the destruction that came with it, as well as making concrete plans to change the trajectory of one's life. These plans include things like learning new skills and establishing a treatment plan. The use of goal setting, self-help manuals, and behavior change techniques are common as is regular counseling while the patient is struggling.

There are medications, both oral and injectable, that can be given to either block the good feelings alcohol causes or exacerbate the bad ones. If you are on one of these medications and try to have a drink, you might end up with nausea, severe vomiting, and headaches as a result. It's like getting a hangover without drinking. Most people, even non-alcoholics, would agree that this takes a lot of the fun out of things.

Other medical treatment possibilities for alcoholism include steps to reverse damage or prevent further damage to the body. Follow-up treatment is focused on support, usually in the form of counseling. Other psychological disorders can be addressed as well, as they are commonly comorbid with alcohol abuse. These include things like anxiety and depression and can commonly be treated with medication and psychotherapy.

The whole idea of follow-up treatment and support is a common one in recovery circles. After any medical intervention has been done, most people are left with cravings, possible light withdrawal symptoms still lingering, and no clue what to do next. Options at this point include group support, such as Alcoholics Anonymous, private therapy, and various behavioral treatments. Each of these has its place, pros and cons, and success rate.

Alcohol recovery in general, no matter the method, has a high relapse rate. Ninety percent of alcoholics will experience at least one relapse in their first four years of sobriety. These relapses can be triggered by anything from a beer advertisement on the side of the road to a period of extreme stress in the alcoholic's life. What the trigger is isn't as important as how the alcoholic handles it. Other common triggers are depression or isolation, both of which could happen as a result of the alcoholic deciding to quit.

Their former drinking buddies may not want to seek them out. Without the social lubricant of alcohol, someone used to drinking may find that they are too anxious to be social. Whatever the reason, an alcoholic who is seeking help must stay aware of their actions in order to not fall into old habits. Though alcohol may not be present or encouraged, a person only gets out of therapy what they are willing to put into it. Sitting down, not sharing or opening up, and leaving early are fine examples of how not to make therapy work for you. Someone who takes an active role in their recovery and gets involved in a support group or finds some other way to openly and safely discuss the struggles of quitting drinking is more likely to give drinking up rather than walk away.

Styles of Recovery Therapy

Psychotherapy, or talk therapy, may be the most common nonmedical treatment for alcoholism. This is encouraged in support groups, 12-step programs, private counseling, and the like. It is thought that the sharing of experiences, symptoms, troubles, and victories can lend a feeling of familiarity as well as reassurance. After all, if one person who had worse habits can cut back on their drinking enough to get a new job, there is nothing stopping you. These methods use mutual encouragement and shared experience to keep people involved and working towards recovery. It is easier to admit to some of the more embarrassing alcohol withdrawal symptoms, like gastrointestinal issues, if you know those you are with have been there too.

Psychotherapy can be practiced in a group setting or one on one. The latter commonly goes more in-depth about any trauma or abuse that might have led to any kind of negative behaviors like alcoholism. It can include practices such as cognitive behavioral therapy. This allows the patient and therapist to reframe negative thinking in order to better process and cope with life's challenges. This goal-oriented style of therapy involves opening up about feelings and learning about resilience and assertiveness.

Dialectical behavior therapy (DBT) is another option that someone can choose. This teaches behavioral skills including mindfulness, or being fully present in the moment. Mindfulness is commonly achieved through focusing exclusively on breathing. Emotional regulation, another common lesson in DBT, teaches how to manage and react to intense emotions when they come. This generally involves lessening a feeling or analyzing a problem with a more calm, logical mindset. Accepting negative emotions rather than escaping them, known as distress tolerance, seems a common method encouraged for alcoholics. Interpersonal effectiveness is the last important step in DBT, where the patient prioritizes themselves and their needs rather than worrying about everyone else in their life.

If sitting around and talking about problems is not your style, you might be helped by experiential therapy. This involves exploring the subconscious and getting in touch with one's own feelings. These practices are also the ones that look the least like traditional therapy. Art therapy, music therapy, and equine therapy are three of the most recognized experiential therapies. On the outside, these practices seem to encourage a patient to open up about their problems through first relaxing and forgetting about them.

The family treatment approach brings in others to help the therapist learn more about the patient. This can be an effective way to know what behaviors could be concerning friends and family of the alcoholic as well as what might need to be addressed. Anger issues or poor financial management may only be known to the alcoholic's spouse, for example. The therapist in family treatment cases will work with the entire group to take care of everyone's needs as the alcoholic recovers. This includes education about the addiction model and teaching coping mechanisms to the entire group.

There are many more therapy types and styles that can help addicts handle and move past their substance abuse. Perhaps one of the most well-known is 12-step facilitation therapy. This is meant to work in conjunction with 12-step rehabilitation groups, like Alcoholics Anonymous. The key ideas of this group include the acceptance of the disease model of addiction, active involvement in group meetings, and the surrender to a higher power with adherence to recovery activities.

There are as many styles of possible therapy as there are people seeking it, but the 12-step programs may be the most well-known and best-publicized in terms of helping with addiction control. These groups tend to be self-led and religiously oriented, but non-denominational and apolitical. The focus is the famed 12 steps meant to guide an addict toward recovery. These steps can be repeated as needed and taken in the order that works best for the individual addict working on them.

The 12 steps include things like admitting to wrongdoing, apologizing, and making up for such actions. After that, people are encouraged to continue with a self-analysis to identify any other wrong action or hurt they gave another. After a sincere apology and some sort of restitution, there is expected to be some sort of spiritual awakening. The addict is encouraged to be a proponent of the 12-step message and tell others about it while turning away from the addiction that caused so much hurt in their lives.

Whatever form of therapy or recovery model might work best for you, it is a good idea to involve other supportive people in your cutting-back process with alcohol. Bringing in others gives you a safe place to talk about your struggles with others who might be able to identify with the situation. Licensed therapists, of course, are required to keep sessions confidential. Friends can be asked to extend the same courtesy if you wish. Therapy gets a bad rap in many circles, but talking openly and honestly about your problems can help you see connections and behavior patterns that may need to be changed.

Help Outside of Therapy

Some people don't want to pour their hearts out to a therapist or even to a friend. They may prefer to deal with problems on their own because the involvement of others has never helped before or has even made things worse. Maybe they don't have health coverage to pay for therapy. In these cases, whatever the reason, there are non-medical and non-therapy solutions that can help ease the difficulties of addiction and substance abuse recovery. Some align with simple good health habits and others encourage a change in attitude for the addict.

Regular exercise is encouraged by many. This can ease some physical symptoms of addiction as well as detoxing. Beginning a regular exercise habit can also provide a distraction from a desire to drink. The endorphins and other feel-good chemicals that flood the brain following a good workout can, over time, replace the buzz of alcohol. As exercise leads to weight loss, better health, and more energy, the alcoholic will likely hear more compliments from those around them. This serves as further encouragement to drink less since alcohol is believed to cause weight gain. Just keep things in moderation. There is no need to get hooked on exercise after letting alcohol go.

Some people like to track their drinking habits. This can be a way of keeping yourself accountable. Making note of how much you drink, how you feel, and what might happen as a result of your drinking gives a tangible log. Being able to look back over these details may remind you why you chose to quit. You can take note of hangovers, drunken injuries, or any other problems that might occur. These can range from minor issues like tripping over furniture to much larger problems like bar fights or sexual assault.

Relaxation techniques are a good distraction method if an alcoholic is tempted to drink. These often involve deep breathing or turning the mind's focus to a specific part of the body. Using these techniques can help calm an alcoholic who once reached for a drink to douse their temper. Getting rid of accumulated stress by relaxing the body's muscles can divert practiced behaviors or habits centered around the physical tension that happens when a person gets angry. Dropping the tension can ease the foul mood and negate the need for alcohol.

Developing a positive attitude and changing one's own mindset takes deliberate action and a lot of awareness. Still, this promises to reprogram triggers that may have already been identified. If an alcoholic has a frustrating family member, someone who "drives them to drink," this is a prime situation for a different mindset. Maybe this person is just enthusiastic about life, ready to share that joy with everyone around them. Now this is the kind of change in mindset that can take time to develop and even more time to accept, but it is still doable. Gaining a more positive mindset may negate reasons to drink for those who are particularly sad or depressed as well.

Learning to let go of the future ties in with the idea of mindfulness, discussed earlier in the book. For an alcoholic to let go of situations they have no control over takes work, but can also eliminate a trigger for some. Many people are driven to drink simply by virtue of their worries over the future. Where is the next paycheck? What is the next meal? Now, the idea of letting go of the future does not mean a total lackadaisical attitude with no planning ahead. Rather, it suggests a lack of overplanning. The only actions any of us can control in this life are our own and worrying beyond that is not always helpful in the long term. By releasing these worries instead of fretting over them, some addicts can lose a reason to drink and find better peace of mind.

Whatever recovery method you choose, allow yourself some growth in the moment. If one method is not working, try another. Maybe you need family therapy with your partner, exercise with a sibling, and cognitive behavioral therapy on your own to make things work. There is no one size fits all, no perfect method that will help everyone cut back on drinking. Find what works for you and adjust what doesn't. Be patient and give yourself time to adapt to changes before rejecting a method or lesson. If you truly want to cut back on your drinking, even if only by a small amount, you will succeed in time.

Chapter 8: Recovery—a Way Forward

"Those who avoid reality mustn't dare counsel others on what reality is nor how it shall be dealt with."—**Daniel V. Chappell**

No matter the reason you started drinking or decided to cut back, taking a serious look at alcohol's effect on your life probably revealed some uncomfortable truths. You may have family or friends begging you to stop. Your bank account might have an alarmingly low balance. Maybe you're functioning well and just have trash bags full of cans to serve as reminders of your addiction. Whatever the case, once you do find the road to recovery, know that it takes time.

Relapses are very common for recovering alcoholics. In fact, they occur for 90% of people in their first four years of quitting. Relapses and withdrawal symptoms are not just felt by those abstaining either. Even a person who is cutting back their intake can feel some of these symptoms. If withdrawal symptoms come, treat the discomfort as best you can. If you experience a relapse, don't beat yourself up over it.

Although that statistic above sounds scary, like the odds are stacked against you, this is not the case. The first year is the hardest, with a 30% relapse rate. In their second year of attempted sobriety, 21% of recovering alcoholics experienced at least one relapse. By the third year, that percentage drops to single digits. Relapses will happen, but all you need to do is accept them and move on.

Take it one day at a time, then one week at a time. If you experience a setback, just remember that tomorrow is another day. One setback will not destroy everything you've done. You will always have a fresh start waiting for you with the next sunrise. Of course, this is an idea that some people struggle with. They may not be used to forgiving themselves or treating themselves with kindness.

While you are recovering from alcohol abuse disorder, it may help to think of yourself as having a chronic health issue. A diabetic has to watch what they eat. In the same way, you have to avoid triggers that may drive you to drink more. This is why giving yourself restrictions can help. If you can only drink a set number of drinks or spend a certain amount of money, you will have more control over the situation. You won't become hopelessly intoxicated. You won't fall back on past habits or bad behaviors.

If you have taken the advice in this book, you have probably found some activities to replace time that was once spent drinking. Feel free to share these activities with family and friends if you wish. They might join you rather than push you to the bar. Your recovery could pave the way for more, with a built-in support group among family and friends. Though this may be wishful thinking, you will never know if you don't try.

Cutting back from alcohol can be an even harder struggle than complete abstinence because the option is still there. You can still drink, within set limitations. This can make an easy excuse to take more than what limits dictate, but that is addiction talking. Making these excuses may, in fact, be a part of your personal addiction pattern. It could be those old habits coming back to get you into more trouble. Do not allow this to happen.

Knowing your triggers, you can either avoid them or completely reframe your thinking around them. Maybe instead of driving down another street to avoid passing the bar, you can find something else on that street that interests you. If you always buy beer from the same store, you can see if they sell other products. This solution may not be for everyone, as it does not limit exposure to former haunts, old habits, or fiends. If you need to avoid your triggers entirely, that is fine and can usually be figured out.

If you are making the effort to recover from alcohol abuse, you need to make sure there is a support network in place. Surround yourself with people who will encourage your efforts and want to see you succeed. Maybe you can get rides to and from your therapy or support group. This kind of gesture can help you by ensuring you get there on time and have no need to deal with the temptation of driving by a bar or some other trigger.

Remember that the friends and family of a person with alcohol abuse syndrome have some of the same rights as the alcoholic. They can also set limits and boundaries around how much they do or don't provide active help to an alcoholic. A spouse may refuse to call in for "sick days" if their partner is sleeping off a hangover. They may refuse to make beer runs, even for the small amounts a recovering alcoholic is allowing themselves. Some people can ask not to be called late at night or at unusual times. This is all okay.

Anyone trying to cut back on their drinking needs to make sure they have a good support system in place. This includes people who can take phone calls at odd hours or for strange reasons. A recovering alcoholic might need to place a call for support at two in the morning because they are being driven crazy by the thought of having a drink and are trying to say no. In a situation like this, it is important that the alcoholic be reminded why they made the choice to cut back or quit.

This is an important key to the reframing of an alcoholic's thinking. If there are important goals in place that will be easier to meet without alcohol in a person's life, those goals need to be kept in view as much as possible. In addition to better health, maybe you want to save money by not buying alcohol. The goal can be made more specific by allotting that money for something. You could save money for a vacation or a new vehicle, perhaps. There are many different options for this and a wide variety of goals that can be set as motivation.

If such motivation is not enough or someone has a different outlook, the focus might need to shift. Some people are motivated by the promise of a reward. Others are drawn in by the fear of failure. For these people, it may be best to have a pros and cons list written up. This could compare the good that alcohol brings to a person's life to the good they will gain if they cut back drinking. Odds are good that cutting back on alcohol will always bring more good than continuing to drink.

With the proper work and care done ahead of time, anyone who is trying to recover from their addictive behaviors can find success. It takes time and a thorough understanding of your personal addiction. You need to know what triggers you, what can be avoided, what can be reframed, and what those undesired behaviors will be replaced with. You can set up a proper support network. Professional therapy is also always available to those who can benefit from it. Whatever you need to do, if you are willing to put in the work, you will succeed.

Everything Changes

Knowing why you want to cut back on your drinking is one important factor to finding success. Another is knowing how you will cut back. Avoidance, reframing thoughts, and recognizing triggers have been addressed, but there are some who need more. Nobody can spend all their time in a support group. For some, it might be better to make a clean break. But why?

Some alcoholics who struggle to find success might need to use more drastic methods. There are many who have skewed perspectives of themselves, their addiction, or the world around them. This distorted worldview is born of an all-or-nothing attitude. Everything is pushed to an extreme in the alcoholic's world. There is no moderation, no middle ground, and no gray area. The presence of these extremes can lead to more of the same.

A completely fresh start is the best solution for some people looking to quit drinking. This means cutting all ties to current behaviors, habits, places, and people. A completely new environment may not eliminate every possible trigger, but can at least negate the familiarity of old habits. There's no worry about the people you used to sit and drink with if they are no longer part of your life. Not living near the bar makes it more difficult to visit regularly.

This method is intended to be a sort of reinvention of the self. People may not be able to uproot their entire lives, but these kinds of extreme methods can be the best way to reframe thoughts and habits. If you can't quit your job, you might be able to move. If you can't move, you can change your driving routes. If you can't do that, you may need to involve some of your support network. For a few days, you might carry cash just to buy lunch from work or gas for your car. If your wallet is at home or in the hands of a partner or trusted friend, you can't spend extra on alcohol.

If you do go to the extreme and reinvent yourself, it may be best to go as far as possible. When a new friend who doesn't know your history suggests a bar visit, you could say you don't drink. If they push, you could say your medications don't allow it. This saves you from going into your entire history and providing a commonly accepted excuse. It may lead to a different destination or give you the role as designated driver. Either way, you are likely to not need to worry about temptation.

Opening up to new people about alcohol addiction and the struggle to recover can give you another source of support, if you choose to do so. You might not want to tell everyone you come across. However, those you do tell each turn into another possible source of support. Maybe you will meet someone who is also trying to stop drinking. You might come across a recovered alcoholic who is further along the recovery road and can mentor you.

Whatever route you choose to take for your own recovery, you need to find something that works for you. Do not try to replicate someone else's journey. Maybe you will reinvent yourself to change the mental image in your head. This is a great way to fight a negative self-image. You aren't a bad person for drinking more than you should. Rather, you are experiencing a personal flaw that you want to move past. Treat yourself kindly and do not take drastic measures unless you have to. Another important thing to do is recognize personal milestones.

Recognize Milestones

Cutting back on alcohol is difficult. There's withdrawal, family complaints, dangers to others, and all the damage done to the body. After deciding to break those habits, you are left to rearrange habits and find ways to remove alcohol from your life. This makes it very important to recognize your successes when they come, no matter how small. This thinking is the reason that Alcoholics Anonymous gives a 24-hour chip to their members. That small step is the first of many.

Giving recognition or celebration to such small milestones might seem silly to some, but it can be very helpful. Looking back to see how far you've come is more effective when there is something significant to see. The steps, milestones, or events that are worth noting can be different for everyone. Some, like the first 24 hours of sobriety, are obviously worth taking note of. There are others that can easily be found if a person wants to look.

The first time an addict reaches out to a friend or family member for help might be worth recognition. This step marks the addict recognizing that they have a problem and they can't solve it entirely on their own. This also marks an official recognition of sorts for the addict's support network. By reaching out for help, the addict is agreeing to use that support. Later actions will determine how often and in what ways the addict might use their network.

Addicts sometimes reach for their supportive friends or family for the wrong reasons. They might lie to get what they want, maybe trying to convince someone to buy alcohol for them. This is not a proper use of a support network. That temptation is too much for some addicts. For this reason, it may be worth recognizing when the addict does not abuse their supportive friends or when they reach out in the right way for the right reasons.

A better way or method for using those supportive people might be something like calling when you feel seriously tempted. You can discuss how you are feeling and might allow the conversation to move to other subjects naturally. This can be important to switch the focus of your thinking. If you call with intention to discuss your desire for alcohol and only discuss that for a long time, it may not help. You will keep the focus on your addiction, meaning you are still thinking about it in the same way you used to. This allows for no reframing of thoughts, no reminders of the negative effects of alcohol, and no reminder of the goals that caused you to cut back on drinking in the first place. If you let the conversation flow freely, after discussing your problems so they are addressed, you may find your way back to healthier behaviors.

Another milestone worth recognizing can be the first time an alcoholic doesn't buy their drink of choice, sometimes called the first drive off. You could celebrate this refusal as a sign that the drink doesn't control them any longer. The thing to remember is that these various milestones and how to celebrate them can be as individualized as needed. In the beginning of the recovery journey, some people need to see a lot of progress and milestones to keep them focused on their goal.

Other milestones can include tracking weight loss, which usually happens early after alcohol intake has been cut down. Nearly everyone can expect to see a few pounds in their first week of less drinking. Timeline milestones are also clear choices: first day, first week, as well as 30, 60, and 90 days. In the first week after abstaining from drinking, alcoholics should get their first good night's sleep with no chemical intervention.

These milestones can be adapted as desired. Maybe someone who drinks with dinner wants to recognize their first meal without alcohol. A person who drinks at bars could celebrate the first time they walk past it. They might decide to celebrate their first time there as a designated driver. You can celebrate any milestone you want in any way you wish.

Milestones can also be celebrated for those who are cutting back rather than abstaining. You could keep a tally and try to go a set number of days only drinking a specific number of drinks. For those who are financially motivated, they could set aside the money normally spent on alcohol and perhaps offer to donate it. This method is not suggested for those whose drinking has ruined their finances. The donation could be to a charity the alcoholic doesn't like with the money getting sent in if any of it is spent on alcohol. This is, again, a drastic method of reframing old habits and not meant for everyone to explore.

All of these milestones are worthy of recognition. There is also no requirement that these happen only once. Setbacks happen during recovery and there is no shame in those. People relapse, mistakes happen. You can pick yourself up and start again. A reset does not negate your previous successes. If you've gone a day without drinking once, you can do it again. Even in setbacks, be sure to celebrate what you do succeed at. You can do this!

Conclusion

"Unless your sober life is more meaningful than your drunk life, you're going to relapse. YOU create the life that matters."—**Toni Sorenson**

Alcohol is one of the most acceptable addictive substances out there, equal to caffeine and nicotine. Many people fall into its grip, and each one has their own reasons for doing so. This can come for any reason. Maybe your finances are in trouble or your family life is no longer calm. Maybe you just want to enjoy better health. No single reason for quitting drinking is any more or less worthy than any other.

Whether quitting or cutting back, you will face challenges that you will need to overcome. These might be self-sabotaging, like buying alcohol you don't need, or might come in the form of friends or family not understanding. The latter is a common issue since alcoholism is so widely accepted. People who don't see problems first-hand tend to forget about them or not think of them. And why not? If a given problem doesn't pose a direct threat or disruption to a specific person, why would they notice? You wasting too much money on beer doesn't affect your neighbor's ability to pay their bills.

If you are a friend or family member of an alcoholic who is trying to recover, you need to be careful how you phrase things around them. Do not ask how long they will be in recovery. Don't act exasperated if they are not making the amount of progress you feel they should be making. If you have agreed to late-night phone calls, be sure not to groan or make comments like "here we go again" as you answer the phone. These sorts of behaviors can trigger negative thoughts and a relapse in your addict. Really, if you are not their therapist, just be supportive and then help to distract. The addict in your life might appreciate the distraction you pose. Follow their lead.

Cutting back on drinking has a great many advantages tied to it, including better physical and mental health. Nobody starts abusing alcohol because things are going well in their lives. These behaviors are more a cry for help. If friends and family know what to watch for, they may be able to encourage early intervention. This may be more wishful thinking than anything, however. Typically, severe alcohol abusers are not noticed until something big happens. An abuse charge, bar fight, or car accident might be the event that prompts family attention.

Between alcohol's wide acceptance in society and people's general tendency to only worry about themselves, the involvement of friends or family in your drinking habits is a fairly positive sign that something needs to change. You may be spending money your family doesn't have. You might be making a fool of yourself. In some extreme cases, your family may even fear you. Whatever the situation, be confident and know that things can change for the better, no matter how things may be now.

Of course, a change for the better may not maintain any of your current habits. There are some alcoholics who need to perform a total overhaul on their lives in order to reach recovery properly. This is a very involved process. Nevertheless, whether you have a foundation set up or are starting from scratch, all addicts face the same obstacles.

Turning away from alcohol, or even cutting back what you drink, can be a challenge. It is important that you remain in control as much as possible. If you choose to set alcohol-free days into your schedule, do not use them as excuses to go crazy the rest of the week. You also need to be entirely honest with yourself about your drinking habits. This will help you know what needs to change and what can stay the same.

Changing habits is not easy for anyone, but there are methods out there to help addicts. If you don't want to drive past a bar you frequent, you can change your route. If you still need to meet with coworkers, you can suggest a different location. If it must be the bar, volunteer to be a designated driver. Every problem has a solution if you are willing to look for it.

Resources Everywhere

A wide variety of resources are out there for people who want to lessen or drop an alcohol addiction. Numerous therapies exist to help with withdrawal symptoms, temptations, and reframing thought processes around alcohol. Many therapists will take health insurance. In extreme cases, a person can be placed in a facility on the word of others. However, this only happens in a situation where the alcoholic poses a tremendous risk to themselves or those around them. The vast majority of alcoholics who have opted to try and recover are not in such a position that they are held against their will.

Learning to work within your addiction and recognizing the signs and triggers that set you off are excellent projects to handle with a trained professional. They can help you identify risk factors, habitual behaviors, and things that might change both. While working through such a plan with your therapist, it is important to be fully open and honest about your situation and your feelings, both physical and emotional. Honesty is key in every recovery.

It is also important to know what kind of therapy you are most comfortable with. Many people like to have one-on-one sessions where they need not fear any judgment in their words. The idea of behavioral therapy also appeals to many since it offers a way to restructure life in a logical cause and effect sort of manner. If I go to the gas station, I'll buy a pack of sodas instead of beer. This sort of replacement behavior can make the act of cutting back easier.

Some people do much better in a group setting. These people tend to rely on the group around them for a sense of accountability. You can tell yourself that you are not attending therapy for yourself. You're going to see how Sam is doing or what Anne might be wearing. Any excuse or reasoning that gets you to attend with a genuinely optimistic attitude will do. Much like the choice to cut back on alcohol, your intention and effort are what count.

Intention, at times, can even be entirely selfish, as long as it works for you. Maybe you keep attending Alcoholics Anonymous meetings just to compare your number of sober days to the person who came in a week after you. This should not be turned into any kind of long-term competition, especially since you are truly only competing against yourself, but if this kind of thinking gets you to put in effort and make changes in the early days, it should be fine. You are the only one who needs to know about this kind of motivation and if it works—it works.

Even if you choose not to go to therapy, that doesn't mean you are completely alone in your efforts. Friends and family who are willing to listen can help. 12-step programs can offer a sense of accountability with like-minded individuals. You can even set up safeguards against yourself by limiting the amount of money you are allowed to spend or the amount of alcohol you are allowed to buy. If you do this, you may choose to share those set limits with a trusted person to provide an extra layer of accountability.

It is important to remember honesty with the self as well as honesty with others. In those interests, a standard drink is 12 ounces of beer, five ounces of wine, or an ounce and a half of hard liquor. Tracking how much you are actually drinking has been known to surprise some people. Tracking can also give you a quick and easy way to mark successes as the number of drinks per day goes down.

Whatever method of treatment you choose to attempt, you can track where you are in that process, which can help some people in seeing progress for their efforts. There are six stages of alcoholic recovery. Each of these stages looks at the relationship between alcohol and the addict. The early stages involve more excuses since the addict is not accepting of their problem yet.

Stage one is known as precontemplation. At this stage, the addict is not likely to attend any treatment without an outside influence. They do not have a problem, are in full control of their drinking, and are fully on the defensive. They are likely experiencing the negative consequences of whatever level of drinking they are at, but may be refusing to admit to having a problem. Alcoholics in this recovery stage often refuse to discuss their addiction openly and will try to redirect conversation. Patience and understanding are the only way to move past this stage.

The involvement of family and friends is crucial in this stage because the alcoholic will only make excuses. People close to them can serve as reminders for reasons to seek help. This can be a difficult balance to strike, but if they can keep the idea of seeking help at the forefront of an alcoholic's mind, that may eventually happen. As long as they do not push the alcoholic further away from the idea that they have a problem, extra involvement can only usher the second stage to come on sooner.

The second stage is contemplation. People in this stage probably recognize they have a problem, but may not see the depth of its severity. Stalling is common at this stage. Yes, the addict will seek help—at some point—in a few months. There is little to no commitment to any firm actions. Many people can stay in this stage of recovery for a long time, not wanting to move forward while they make excuses for their drinking and negate the severity of their problem.

Contemplation can be a difficult stage for those close to the alcoholic. Seeing the problem and seeing how bad it is are not the same thing. Here, again, reminders can help but also may hurt. There is always a balance to strike with alcoholics. Coming on too strongly can seem like an attack, but a weak approach can easily be brushed off as unimportant. Communication is key, which is why tools like group or family therapy can help so much.

Stage three is known as preparation. At this point, the addict is committed to making a change for the better. Planning is crucial to this stage. The addict needs to take time, look at their behaviors, and plan specific alternative behaviors to keep from falling back on old habits. Addicts who skip this crucial planning stage are more likely to fail without a set of actionable steps in hand. This stage can last for up to 18 months. It involves all of the behavior changes and avoiding triggers that have been previously discussed.

This stage may be one where the addition of others can do more harm than good. The addict knows their situation, their addiction, and their mind the best. They need to work out for themselves what plans can be carried out, how to cut back, and what to do when temptation hits the hardest. Having someone point out the struggles they have with an addiction they are not experiencing or trying to cut down can only add unnecessary work and burdens to the alcoholic. There is no need, yet, for a full reform of every aspect of the alcoholic's life. Small steps are both necessary and important.

Maintenance is the fifth stage. This is where all the plans and new behaviors slowly become second nature. Adopting healthy coping strategies and finding new hobbies are both keys to this stage. As the addict develops past their addiction, they can enjoy the benefits of sobriety. This is also when organ damage begins to repair itself, provided the addict has been abstaining long enough.

In this stage, the involvement of others can go back to being a huge help. If the addict has a good handle on their new behaviors, there is no need to worry over major relapses. Friends and family do need to remember that relapses happen at any stage and should be forgiven with encouragement offered to hit the reset button and start again. Pointing out sobriety benefits or subtler gestures like spending more time around the addict the less they drink can help drive home the reasons for cutting back on alcohol. These reminders can be very encouraging when an alcoholic looks back to see how far they have come in their recovery journey.

The final stage is known as termination and there are many theories surrounding it. Some people say alcohol addiction is a lifelong problem, citing evidence as addicts show some of the same behaviors even without alcohol in their system. This is known as dry drunk and involves behaviors such as impulsivity and dysfunctionality. Some people argue that the presence of these behaviors proves that the problem of alcoholism never truly leaves. Despite this attitude, technically, at this stage, the addict has no further desire for alcohol and is therefore completely cured.

Impulsive and dysfunctional behaviors are the thing to watch for here. Someone with an addictive personality or a genetic predisposition for alcohol abuse might go from cutting back on booze to finding some other vice. Gambling, smoking, or illegal drugs are just a few possibilities. Impulsive behaviors for recovering alcoholics can include unnecessary spending, unhealthy snap decisions, or things like adopting a new vice. Even something healthy, like exercise, can become damaging if it is not practiced in moderation. A lack of moderation truly defines the structure and format of an alcohol abuser's life, but this does not have to be forever.

To a Brighter Future

Cutting back on alcohol may be a challenge, but everyone has some reason that will keep them trying. The promise of extra money, better health, and a more peaceful homelife might be what keeps you motivated. Drinking less can improve your career prospects as well. Even something as simple as no hangovers in the morning or a night of peaceful sleep can be enough of a draw. Whatever reason drives you to put in the effort is good enough.

Spread the word about what you are doing. Tell family and friends. Build your support network early so that anyone who may be troublesome can reveal themselves. If you have a friend who says they will support your attempts to cut back on alcohol, but then they offer to buy every other round or come to your house with a 12 pack in hand, that is not someone you need in your support network. Either point out how their actions are hurting you and ask if they are willing to change or cut contact for a time as much as you are able. This may seem like a harsh conclusion, but adding extra sources of temptation will only make things harder for you.

Communicate your needs clearly with those around you. If there are specific dry nights where you need no alcohol, you might ask family members or frequent household visitors to join you. Planning some activities can stave off temptation; a family game night or a walk around the neighborhood can take your mind off of your struggles. You might also find that your family is happy to spend time with a more sober you.

Try to remember that your family is on this search with you, everyone trying to figure out how a life with less alcohol works. They may want to open up to you about their feelings around your drinking. Only do this under the supervision of a trained therapist or when you feel completely ready to deal with the outcome, especially in the early days. If a family member or friend wants to talk, give them that opportunity, but do not feel like you have to shoulder their burdens as well as your own. If the discussion gets too triggering or bothers you too much, you have every right to excuse yourself. Maybe suggest someone else they can talk to, like another friend who can sympathize with their struggles.

As a recovering alcoholic, you need to prioritize your own care first. If you need those dry days, take them and don't feel bad about it. If you need to attend therapy twice a month, do it and be open and honest about all you are experiencing. If you need to sit in a convenience store parking lot for 10 minutes, debating about whether to go in and buy alcohol, do it and be proud of yourself when you drive off empty-handed. Make sure your needs are met.

Getting to a healthier place, mentally speaking, can lead you to bigger and better things slowly. In fact, the improvements of mental and physical health are inextricably linked. Feeling healthier gives you more energy, which, in turn, leads to more endorphins in the brain and better moods overall. All of this is a process of slow growth. What may start with two fewer beers a week may grow into a reduction to six beers. Attending support groups can give you more contact with people who are facing the same struggles. One day, you may even find yourself in a mentor position, helping some other people who are seeking their own recovery.

This particular goal may not be for everyone, but sometimes these things work themselves out. You may set out just to eliminate one six pack per week from what you normally drink. As you cut down your regular drinks one glass or can at a time, your body begins to feel the effects. Fewer hangovers, fewer headaches, and less damage to your brain are just the beginning when compared to where you might end up. After you eliminate your first regular six pack, you might run into someone else in the middle of their own struggle. If you can reach out and help them, offer your input and experiences, then you may be one more motivator. You might keep cutting back on alcohol to show someone else they can do the same thing.

Remember that everyone has their own motivations and what draws you in may not apply to someone else's situation. Do not let another person's setback affect you and don't let yourself fall off the wagon because of somebody else's success. Just keep your goals in sight and try not to let temptation draw you in too often. Forgive setbacks and allow yourself to get up and try again.

Turning away from alcohol in any measure may be one of the biggest challenges and greatest triumphs of your life. Celebrate those victories, no matter how small. Keep careful logs so that you can look back and see how far you've come. You can become a better person by beating addiction. Remember that you can control your alcohol consumption. It does not need to control you.

References

"Alcohol Addiction Recovery Methods - 12 Step & Non 12 Step." Alcohol Abuse, www.alcoholabuse.com/recovery/recovery-methods/. Accessed 26 Sept. 2021.

"Alcohol Relapse Rates and Statistics." The Recovery Village Drug and Alcohol Rehab, 6 Dec. 2017, www.therecoveryvillage.com/alcohol-abuse/related-topics/alcohol-relapse-statistics/.

"Alcohol Use Disorder - Diagnosis and Treatment - Mayo Clinic." Www.mayoclinic.org, www.mayoclinic.org/diseases-conditions/alcohol-use-disorder/diagnosis-treatment/drc-20369250#:~:text=But%20if%20used%20in%20addition%20to%20your%20treatment. Accessed 26 Sept. 2021.

"Alcohol Withdrawal Symptoms, Detox Timeline & Treatment." American Addiction Centers, American Addiction Centers, 2019, americanaddictioncenters.org/withdrawal-timelines-treatments/alcohol.

"Alcohol Withdrawal Timeline: Signs, Symptoms & Detox Process." Recovery First Treatment Center, recoveryfirst.org/alcohol-abuse/withdrawal-timeline/. Accessed 26 Sept. 2021.

"Alcoholic Recovery Stages." Drug Rehab, 17 Jan. 2018, www.drugrehab.com/addiction/alcohol/stages-of-recovery/.

"Alcoholism Statistics & Information on Group Demographics." Alcohol.org, 2019, www.alcohol.org/statistics-information/.

"Alcohol's Effects on the Body | National Institute on Alcohol Abuse and Alcoholism (NIAAA)." Www.niaaa.nih.gov, www.niaaa.nih.gov/alcohols-effects-health/alcohols-effects-body#:~:text=Here%E2%80%99s%20how%20alcohol%20can%20affect%20your%20body%3A%20Alcohol. Accessed 26 Sept. 2021.

Brown, Nicole. "How Much Money Do Alcoholics Actually Spend on Alcohol? | ATA." Addicted to Alcohol, 27 Feb. 2018, addictedtoalcohol.com/information/money-alcoholics-spend-alcohol/.

CDC. "CDC - Fact Sheets-Alcohol Use and Health - Alcohol." Centers for Disease Control and Prevention, 2018, www.cdc.gov/alcohol/fact-sheets/alcohol-use.htm.

FastStats - Alcohol Use. 2019, www.cdc.gov/nchs/fastats/alcohol.htm.

Fitzgerald, Kelly. "Why Alcohol Is the Deadliest Drug - Addiction Center." AddictionCenter, 13 Dec. 2017, www.addictioncenter.com/community/why-alcohol-is-the-deadliest-drug/.

https://www.facebook.com/WebMD. "Food Calorie Counter & Calculator." WebMD, 2018, www.webmd.com/diet/healthtool-food-calorie-counter.

—. "Slideshow: What Does Alcohol Do to Your Body?" WebMD, 2018, www.webmd.com/mental-health/addiction/ss/slideshow-alcohol-body-effects.

Huett, Kayla. "Treatment Methods & Evidence-Based Practices." National Association of Addiction Treatment Providers, 24 Aug. 2020, www.naatp.org/addiction-treatment-resources/treatment-methods.

"If You Quit Drinking, You May Experience These Withdrawal Symptoms." Verywell Mind, www.verywellmind.com/symptoms-of-alcohol-withdrawal-63791.

Kovacs, Jenny Stamos. "The Dos and Don'ts of Counting Calories." WebMD, www.webmd.com/diet/features/dos-donts-counting-calories#1.

National Institute on Alcohol Abuse and Alcoholism. "Alcohol Facts and Statistics." National Institute of Alcohol Abuse and Alcoholism, 26 June 2019, www.niaaa.nih.gov/publications/brochures-and-fact-sheets/alcohol-facts-and-statistics.

—. "Treatment for Alcohol Problems: Finding and Getting Help | National Institute on Alcohol Abuse and Alcoholism (NIAAA)." Nih.gov, 2017, www.niaaa.nih.gov/publications/brochures-and-fact-sheets/treatment-alcohol-problems-finding-and-getting-help.

NIAAA. "Underage Drinking | National Institute on Alcohol Abuse and Alcoholism (NIAAA)." Nih.gov, 2017, www.niaaa.nih.gov/publications/brochures-and-fact-sheets/underage-drinking.

Robinson, Katie. "Best Drinking Quotes to Help Curb Alcohol Abuse." EverydayHealth.com, 17 Apr. 2018, www.everydayhealth.com/alcoholism/living-with/best-drinking-quotes-help-alcohol-addiction/.

September 25, Editorial StaffUpdated: "Dealing with Difficult People in Alcoholics Anonymous -." Alcoholrehab.com, alcoholrehab.com/alcohol-recovery/dealing-with-difficult-people-in-alcoholics-anonymous/. Accessed 26 Sept. 2021.

"Signs of Alcoholism: Symptoms of Early, Chronic & End Stages." American Addiction Centers, 2019, americanaddictioncenters.org/alcoholism-treatment/stages.

"The Five Types of Alcoholics." Drug Rehab, 9 Jan. 2018, www.drugrehab.com/addiction/alcohol/types-of-alcoholics/. Accessed 26 Sept. 2021.

"The No BS Guide to Setting Healthy Boundaries in Real Life." Healthline, 10 Dec. 2018, www.healthline.com/health/mental-health/set-boundaries#affirming-boundaries.

Thomas, Scott. "The Effects of Alcohol on the Body." American Addiction Centers, 2019, americanaddictioncenters.org/alcoholism-treatment/body-effects.

Watkins, Meredith. "What Are the Problems & Effects of Alcoholism on Families & Marriages." American Addiction Centers, 2021, americanaddictioncenters.org/alcoholism-treatment/family-marital-problems.

"What People Recovering from Alcoholism Need to Know about Osteoporosis | NIH Osteoporosis and Related Bone Diseases National Resource Center."

Bones.nih.gov, bones.nih.gov/health-info/bone/osteoporosis/conditions-behaviors/alcoholism. Accessed 26 Sept. 2021.

"Which Household Products Contain Alcohol?" Alcohol.org, www.alcohol.org/alcoholism/household-products-abuse/#:~:text=If%20you%20consume%20these%20household%20items%2C%20even%20in. Accessed 26 Sept. 2021.

Printed in Great Britain
by Amazon

74410900R00059